THE EVERYTHING®
Running Book
2nd Edition

Dear Reader,

Believe it or not, I didn't begin running until I was nearly thirty years old. If someone had told me when I was a teenager that I would become a runner, what's more, a marathoner, I would have said he was insane! In high school I couldn't even make it around the quarter-mile track without gasping for air. I started running as part of a lifestyle change and soon after realized how much I enjoyed my newfound sport.

In 1983, after a year of running, I completed my first 26.2 mile (marathon) race, finishing in 3 hours and 24 minutes (3:24). I've since run twenty marathons in nineteen different states, with a personal best of 3:11. My running experiences have led to a variety of coaching opportunities at the high school and college level and with the Leukemia and Lymphoma Society's Team in Training program. Through my Web site, *www.marathontraining.com*, I provide personal training services to runners throughout the United States and the world.

The message I offer to anyone considering beginning a running program is simple: If I can do it, you can too! You'll find that once you start running, your overall health and energy level will improve and you'll experience a more positive outlook on life. Whether you're a beginner training for your first 5K race or an experienced runner trying to improve upon your previous marathon time, *The Everything® Running Book, 2nd Edition* provides comprehensive training information on a wide range of running-related topics. It is your all-in-one training resource—and running companion. Welcome to the wonderful world of running!

Art Liberman

Welcome to the EVERYTHING® Series!

These handy, accessible books give you all you need to tackle a difficult project, gain a new hobby, comprehend a fascinating topic, prepare for an exam, or even brush up on something you learned back in school but have since forgotten.

You can read an *Everything*® book from cover to cover or just pick out the information you want from our four useful boxes: e-questions, e-facts, e-alerts, e-ssentials. We give you everything you need to know on the subject, but throw in a lot of fun stuff along the way, too.

We now have more than 400 *Everything*® books in print, spanning such wide-ranging categories as weddings, pregnancy, cooking, music instruction, foreign language, crafts, pets, New Age, and so much more. When you're done reading them all, you can finally say you know *Everything*®!

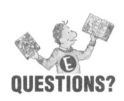

QUESTIONS?
Answers to common questions

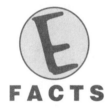

FACTS
Important snippets of information

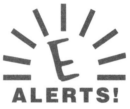

ALERTS!
Urgent warnings

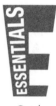

ESSENTIALS
Quick handy tips

Editorial

Director of Innovation: Paula Munier

Editorial Director: Laura M. Daly

Executive Editor, Series Books: Brielle K. Matson

Associate Copy Chief: Sheila Zwiebel

Acquisitions Editor: Kerry Smith

Development Editor: Brett Palana-Shanahan

Production Editor: Casey Ebert

Production

Director of Manufacturing: Susan Beale

Production Project Manager: Michelle Roy Kelly

Prepress: Erick DaCosta, Matt LeBlanc

Design Manager: Heather Blank

Interior Layout: Heather Barrett, Brewster Brownville, Colleen Cunningham

Visit the entire Everything® series at www.everything.com

THE
EVERYTHING®
RUNNING
BOOK

2nd Edition

From circling the block to completing
a marathon, training and techniques to
make you a better runner

Art Liberman
Founder, MarathonTraining.com

with Stephen Pribut, D.P.M., and Carlo De Vito

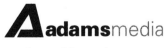
Adamsmedia

Avon, Massachusetts

This book is dedicated to Dr. George Sheehan and to Dr. Charlie Post. Although they are no longer with us, each inspired me greatly while teaching me so much about the relationship and delicate balance between running and life.

An Everything® Series Book.
Everything® and everything.com® are registered trademarks of F+W Publications, Inc.

Published by Adams Media, an F+W Publications Company
57 Littlefield Street, Avon, MA 02322 U.S.A.
www.adamsmedia.com

ISBN 10: 1-59869-506-1
ISBN 13: 978-1-59869-506-9

Printed in the United States of America.

J   I   H   G   F   E   D   C   B

Library of Congress Cataloging-in-Publication Data
available from the publisher.

Disclaimer: The exercise program within *The Everything® Running Book* or any other exercise program may result in injury. Consult your doctor before beginning this or any exercise program. If you begin to feel faint or dizzy while doing any of the exercises in this book, consult your doctor.

This publication is designed to provide accurate and authoritative information with regard to the subject matter covered. It is sold with the understanding that the publisher is not engaged in rendering legal, accounting, or other professional advice. If legal advice or other expert assistance is required, the services of a competent professional person should be sought.

—From a *Declaration of Principles* jointly adopted by a Committee of the American Bar Association and a Committee of Publishers and Associations

Many of the designations used by manufacturers and sellers to distinguish their products are claimed as trademarks. Where those designations appear in this book and Adams Media was aware of a trademark claim, the designations have been printed with initial capital letters.

This book is available at quantity discounts for bulk purchases.
For information, please call 1-800-289-0963.

Contents

Acknowledgments

My acknowledgements begin with happy memories of my mom, Sylvia, and brother, Jack, who passed away in 1988 and 1995, respectively. They both took the time to listen, care, and exemplify how to live a good life. They also emphasized the importance of giving oneself to others. Thanks also to my father, Sam, and brother, Robert, who helped me develop a strong work ethic and passion toward my career and personal interests while demonstrating to me in their own ways how to strive for and attain excellence in all that I undertake.

I owe much gratitude to my first running mentors, Dr. Brian Smith and Terry Hamlin, for imparting to me, both as a runner and as a coach, many of the training methods and philosophies that I use today. Thanks also to Randy Brown, my personal friend and fellow coach, for helping me further refine my coaching skills. I have appreciated his counsel and support over the years, and also with this project.

Thanks to all the runners I've had the pleasure to train with and coach over the past twenty-five years, including those with the Leukemia and Lymphoma Society's Team in Training program, members of the cross-country teams at the College of Charleston and North Charleston High School, and visitors/clients of my Web site, "State of the Art Marathon Training" (*www.marathontraining.com*). You've all taught me more about running and coaching than you can imagine!

Thanks to Dominique and Carlo DeVito and Dr. Stephen Pribut for their editorial assistance, journalistic contribution, and support with this book. You guys were great!

Enjoy *The Everything® Running Book, 2nd Edition*, and I'll see you on the roads!

—Art Liberman

Top Ten Reasons to Run

1. Physical fitness: You'll lower your resting heart rate, strengthen your heart, improve your cardiovascular system, strengthen and tone your muscles, and increase bone density.

2. If you want to lose weight and body fat, running will help.

3. Runner's High. This is the elevated mood you get when you are running "in the zone," or when you come off a particularly inspiring workout.

4. Running is one of the easiest, most convenient forms of exercise.

5. Running is a sport that you can do either by yourself or with others.

6. Running alone is a meditative activity. You'll find yourself solving problems that have been pestering you, gaining insight into your life, and just plain feeling better about life.

7. Running with others is a good bonding exercise and can be a friendship-building experience.

8. Running is accessible to almost everyone, from kids to senior citizens.

9. You *and* your dog need more exercise. When both of you start easy and build up, you become a fitness team!

10. Running helps you see the world. No matter where you travel, so long as you have your running shoes and the proper clothes, you can find a place to run. You'll observe things you would never notice any other way, and you'll feel more a part of your locale.

Introduction

▶ WHY RUN? Running is an exercise available to almost all people. And it also has one of the lowest equipment needs of any sport. You don't need a ball, a field, or an umpire. You don't need a gym, a pool, or a track. You might already own everything you need: running shoes, a T-shirt, and a pair of shorts. That's about it.

Sure, there are runners who go beyond the basics. As with other competitive sports, runners make use of gadgets like GPS speedometers, fancy warm-up suits, and elaborate heart rate monitors. However, these aren't essential items for the beginner or novice runner. (The difference between beginner and novice runners is discussed in Chapter 11.)

Another benefit is that you can run alone or with other people. You might run with friends at the same pace or else run with them competitively. You can choose to run with one person or with a large group. Running is good for the whole family. All ages are encouraged to participate and compete.

And there are runners everywhere. Going on a trip? There are runners all over the United States, Europe, Australia, and South America. Just name a locale, and there is sure to be a local running club. Don't know where to go for your next vacation? How about a 5K race in Charleston, South Carolina or a 5-miler in Chicago? Try a marathon in New York, Boston, Los Angeles, or Hawaii. There are thousands of road races held each year in vacation spots all over the United States and the world, from the 5K to marathons.

The point is that runners are everywhere. And everyone who runs is a runner. Even the man or woman who finishes last in a 5K or a marathon is still called a runner. How fast you run is not necessarily a yardstick by which other runners will judge you. In running, it's not you versus the other person. The supreme fascination of running is that it is you against you!

Beginning a running program offers numerous benefits, not least of which is your health. For every hour you run 10-minute miles, you burn 4.2 calories per body pound. Jumping rope burns 3.8 calories per body pound and swimming 3.5 calories per body pound. Half an hour spent running is comparable to riding a bike for an hour, chopping wood for an hour, playing tennis doubles, or weight training for an hour. Compared with other fitness activities, the benefits of running provide a timesaving advantage in a fast-paced world.

Take it from Ed Daley of Freehold, New Jersey: "I began running in 1979. It enabled me to keep my weight down and it improved my quality of life. I enjoyed life more, I wasn't tired, wasn't heavy. I was able to do more things with ease and comfort. Running improved my fitness and my outlook. I felt better about everything."

In this book you'll learn how to stay on track and become motivated enough to get to the point where you don't want to miss a run There's also lots of important running-related health and nutritional information as well. Many folks shy away from learning about physical fitness because they think it is complicated, but this book simplifies the subject for you. Your running will benefit from your increased expertise.

Find out for yourself about the new healthier lifestyle that awaits you. It costs pennies a day and will make a huge impact on your life. The latter is the best reason of all to start. Enjoy, and good luck!

Chapter 1

Try It, You'll Like It!

As labor-saving advances such as dishwashers, automobiles, and riding mowers have changed people's lifestyles, humans have lost something valuable: regular physical work. Because people have now mechanized even simple activities that use their arms, legs, back, heart, and lungs, their bodies have become correspondingly more flaccid, fat, and weak. People are meant to be active, so much so that their very health depends upon it. Running is one way to help your body thrive.

Striving for Physical Fitness

Personal fitness is not a destination that you visit occasionally in life. Rather, fitness is the actual journey, an ongoing state of health. Participating regularly in a fitness program ensures your best chance of an improved quality and length of life.

So how do you become fit? As with any project, when you use the right tools the job is much more productive, efficient, and even fun. The tools for fitness include exercise and nutrition. In this book, running is the exercise of choice. But to get started, you need to begin where all activity originates—in the mind.

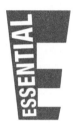

Take a minute to write down five reasons why you want to get fit through incorporating running in your life. You may be surprised by your reasons, which in turn might change over time. Review your answers in one month, then two, to see your progress.

Getting in the Right Mindset

It may seem contradictory, but in fact physical fitness really does begin in the mind. In order for your body to get moving, you need the right mindset. Common reasons people give for not running are discussed next. How many do you recognize as ones you've used yourself?

You Don't Have Enough Time

You might think, "I don't have time to run" or "Running is not the most important thing I need to do today." However, you have a choice about how to spend your time. Ask yourself what is the most important thing you need to do today. What is it that you are making time for? Is your health important to you? Keep in mind that of the most effective exercise options, running requires the least amount of time.

You're Worried about How You'll Look

You may also be concerned with how you'll look while running, even worrying that you'll look silly. If you think everyone else who runs looks silly, too, you'll be in good company at least! When you're fit and feeling good, though, you won't look or feel silly. Similarly, you might dislike the prospect of sweating a lot when you run. Just remember that sweating is a natural bodily function, and you'll be glad to have a working cooling system.

You Don't Want to Get Hurt

If you're afraid you'll hurt yourself running, read on. You'll learn exactly how to take care of yourself in this book. When performed properly, running should be neither uncomfortable nor painful. You'll learn how to run safely and systematically so that you achieve a level of fitness that results in a healthier lifestyle than the one you are currently engaging in. Finally, don't be concerned that you're too old to run. That is the mindset of your old life. Start your new life today. No one is too old to run.

You Don't Want to Spend the Money

Perhaps you are concerned that running is expensive and has hidden costs. However, running is probably the most inexpensive form of exercise. Moreover, being unhealthy is expensive in the long run.

No More Excuses: Time for the New You

There are always excuses for not doing what you really want to do. You probably recognize from the preceding section reasons you've given in the past not to run. Now is the time to stop making excuses. To get yourself ready to be a runner, you need a new way of thinking about running.

Adjust Your Attitude

First, let go of preconceived ideas about fitness and running. Acknowledge and release old negative attitudes. These are unhealthy roadblocks, no longer useful to you. You have a choice regarding what you think about, so let those negative thoughts go and start anew.

Maybe you think you will never enjoy running. Think instead about the benefits it provides: new friends, improved energy, a better mood, and healthier lifestyle. As with most new runners who persevere, you will probably come to love running if you just give it a chance.

The best way to approach running is through an adventurous spirit. When was the last time you tried something new and healthy? Challenge yourself; be a risk taker. And if nothing else works to motivate you, think of the phrase that Nike made famous: "Just do it!"

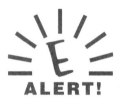

Build a solid relationship with running. You don't start running by doing a marathon. Set short workouts as a goal, and be proud of what you accomplish. Learn by taking small steps, and your relationship with running (or walking/running) will become a lifelong love affair.

Make Time to Run

Think of running as a daily, non-negotiable activity. Do you think about whether or not you are going to brush your teeth each day? Your dental hygiene is a non-negotiable part of your routine that you wouldn't think of not doing. That is how you should begin thinking about running. It is a routine to fit into your day.

Consider time spent running as keeping a health appointment with yourself. If you suffered a life-challenging illness but through regular treatments could reclaim your health, wouldn't you plan your time to go to those appointments? Well, running is a life-saving appointment! It helps prevent a variety of sedentary-based conditions, such as cardiovascular disease.

Build a Relationship with Running

Becoming a runner will take more than a short-term commitment. Add running to your life as you would build a long-term relationship: day in, day out Start out dating, go slowly, and take some time to get to know yourself as a runner.

Focus on the Health Benefits of Running

Turn your view of health inside out. How much time do you spend tending to your exterior appearance, concerned with clothes, hair, nails, and skin? Many people spend more time attending to their exterior appearance than to their interior health. The truth is, your outer appearance depends on your underlying health. Next time you look in the mirror, look more deeply at your body. Imagine how running will improve both the appearance and inner health of your body. Which looks better—a new piece of clothing or the way your clothes fit after you've lost 5–15 percent of your body fat?

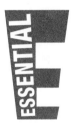

"Being an emergency physician, I encounter my share of stressful days (and nights). I have consistently found, however, that I feel better, perform better, and am actually a more empathetic doctor when I work after running. I am convinced of a neurohormonal response that takes place in my body and which energizes me, yet at the same time settles me and helps me focus, even under harried circumstances."—Ben Bobrow, Las Vegas, NV

Think of your running time as an investment in your health that yields invaluable returns. Through only one half-hour a day (that's less than 2 percent of your whole day!), you can reap the rewards. You—not other market conditions—control this investment. Regular running is vital to achieving optimal health while also helping to protect you from many preventable diseases. Running costs can be less expensive than what you pay for most life insurance policies, and you realize the benefits while you are still alive.

Talk to Other Runners

If you ask runners how they feel after including regular exercise in their lives, would you expect them to say any of the following?

- Running makes me feel lethargic, grouchy, and stressed.
- Running makes me feel worse about myself.
- Running makes me feel and look terrible in my clothes.
- Running makes me fatter.
- Running makes my sleep pattern poorer.
- Running made me start smoking and drinking.
- Running makes my blood pressure go up.

Of course not! You probably know that people who run regularly claim just the opposite. They boast renewed energy, a better outlook on life, a tendency to eat healthier foods, better quality of sleep, and more. What is it about running that produces such effects? It's the fact that running is a form of aerobic exercise.

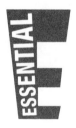

If your friends are runners already, ask them what they like and dislike about running. If they're not runners, ask whether they'd like to be. Recruit one of your nonrunning friends to start a running program with you and share experiences as you train. You'll double your pleasure as well as be able to share your challenges.

Aerobic exercise does for the body what no other activity can because of a crucial process: the utilization of oxygen. You take in oxygen all the time just by breathing, of course. But when you run, you take in greater amounts of oxygen, and it is delivered more deeply into the body because the heart, lungs, and muscles are working harder. Circulation increases and with it, oxygen delivery. This is beneficial for your body and makes you feel good.

The body loves regular bouts of oxygen-rich running and like a welcome houseguest makes accommodations for this. The body actually craves a higher aerobic level. The accommodations are the training benefits that improve the working of the body not only during exercise but also while at rest. No wonder exercise makes us feel better.

Benefits of Running

It is highly motivating to know that you are improving yourself on the inside and the outside. Following are some common and well-documented physiological benefits of running. Let's take a look at what's awaiting you.

Physical Benefits of Running

Running helps to improve respiration, making you an "easy breather." When you run, your body needs more oxygen to fund the activity. Your lungs work harder than when they are at rest to supply the extra demand for oxygen to the body. With repetition over time, your lungs adapt to the extra workload and become more efficient at providing the extra oxygen needed for the activity. The overall effect of this extra work is that you experience more efficient and easier breathing at rest as well as when you are active.

Running also improves cardiac output. Just as success can be measured in terms of productivity or output, cardiac output refers to the productivity of the heart. It is a measure of heart rate and volume of blood pumped out with each heartbeat. When you run, your heart beats at a much faster rate than when you are at rest so that your muscles receive more blood. The more you run, the stronger and more efficient your heart becomes. The training effect of running upon cardiac output is such that the heart at rest beats slowly yet is able to pump large amounts of blood with each beat. You get more output for less effort, improving your heart's efficiency.

As with cardiac output, running also positively affects the vascular system. Blood and oxygen move through the vascular system, the body's highway. As a result of running, veins and arteries become cleaner due to a reduction of fatty deposits. Exercise also increases the number and size of blood vessels, which is the equivalent of more paved streets in your neighborhood making travel less congested and less laborious. The effect is to improve your circulation and blood pressure.

An additional benefit of running occurs with improved muscular strength and endurance. When you run, you use one of the body's major tools: its muscles. You need muscular strength and endurance in order to perform activity or work. Muscular endurance means your ability to maintain activity or work over time. One of the effects of running is to keep your muscles functional and strong.

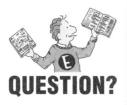

QUESTION?

What is meant by the "training effect"?
The training effect refers to your body's response to a workout. When your body is stressed by exercise, it makes physical adaptations afterward so it won't be as stressed during future workouts. These positive changes you associate with exercise are the training effects.

Running also contributes to increased bone density. Muscles are attached to bone, so when you move your muscles during running, it is as if the muscles are massaging and tugging on the bones. The training effect upon your bones has to do with growth. Think of muscular movement like a bone massage that stimulates bone growth. Bone growth helps to keep bones dense, firm, and healthy.

In addition to stimulating bone growth, running can also improve the flexibility of your joints. A joint is the place where bones meet. Movement of your joints feels good; lack of joint movement feels bad. The training effect on your joints from running will improve their mobility.

Another benefit of running you might be unfamiliar with is an improvement in bowel function. Running helps to stimulate the wavelike movement in the bowels called peristalsis. This happens in part through pressure changes inside the body as a result of increased breathing. Regular and easy elimination prevents hemorrhoids and constipation.

Another physical benefit of running is enhanced sensory motor skills. As a baby and youngster you learned how to use your sensory skills; you learned about balance and movement in space through activity. In order to keep these sensory skills sharp, you have to use them. A training effect of running is the maintenance and improvement of sensory skills, like balance and movement through space or from place to place.

Psychological Benefits of Running

A well-known training effect of running is the production of endorphins. Endorphins are natural morphine-like hormones that produce a sense of well-being and reduce stress levels. They make you feel good and improve your mood. You may have heard of the "runner's high" associated with long-distance runners, but this group doesn't have exclusive rights to endorphin production. You, too, can produce your own endorphins through regular running exercise.

Another psychological benefit is that running fosters creativity and problem-solving ability in many people. Frequently runners use their daily run as a time to reflect, plan their days, and clear their minds from the pressures of a hectic workday.

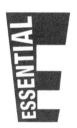

"I began running in June of 2000 at a time in my life when I was very depressed and overweight. I knew I had to do something to make my life better. I began running and it changed my life. Since I began running, I have lost 55 pounds and my self-esteem and self-confidence levels are very high."—Danielle Utillo, Staten Island, NY

Social Benefits of Running

People are social animals who enjoy and need human interaction. Running builds self-confidence, which spreads to other aspects of your life. Don't be surprised if you feel a bit more outgoing and sociable after beginning your running program; this is another training effect of exercise.

Opportunities for social interaction present themselves indirectly as well as directly. You might directly choose to run with others. But even if you prefer running as a time for yourself, you can still indirectly use the subject as a conversation piece in other social situations.

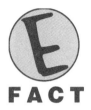

FACT

"Camaraderie is one of the main benefits of joining a running club. It gives you the opportunity to socialize and meet other runners. You exchange information, pick up running tips, maybe even find a training partner."—Linda Hyer, Marlboro, NJ, former president of the Freehold Area Running Club

Your loved ones will be proud of you for your commitment to running. Suppose someone special says to you, "I started a running program a month ago." Do you reply, "Oh no, how could you do such a thing?" or "Oh, I'm so sorry"? Of course not. You probably congratulate him or her and offer support. Others will have the same reaction toward you, helping to reinforce your motivation.

You Will Feel Better, Absolutely!

If you could achieve the psychological benefits discussed in this chapter without exercise, say through medical and therapeutic services instead, you would have to spend numerous hours and large sums of money, take various medications, and likely deal with some negative side effects. In addition, you would not have much fun in the process, and there are no guarantees that the medical and therapeutic means would work. Running can make you feel better with less expense, less stress, and more enjoyment. So now that you have a more positive mindset about running, it's time to learn how to be successful in this new undertaking.

Chapter 2

Setting Yourself Up for Success

Before you trot off to create the new you, there are some basic things you need to know to protect yourself over time. After all, this is not going to be just another hobby started and given up. It's going to become your way of life. The fact that you are reading this book indicates your seriousness about this new sport. Let these pages be your source of information and inspiration as you begin your running program.

Getting Specific about Running Goals

In order to come up with a program that will work best for you, you need to be specific about your needs and goals. Obtain a new notebook and label it simply "Running." On the first page, think about what you want to accomplish. Consider, for example:

- Is your primary goal to lose a certain amount of weight? How much do you want to lose? Be realistic about how long it should take. You'll have a sense of how well the running compliments the other work you do to reach your weight-loss goal once you are doing it regularly. Don't assume, however, that a slow mile-long jog every few days is going to drop you from a size 10 to a size 6 in a couple of months. Jogging will certainly help to lose inches, but it'll take time.
- Is your goal to advance from an occasional run through the neighborhood park to competing in an organized race? Do you want to start with a 5K, or have you suddenly decided you want to run a marathon next year?
- Have you chosen running as an economical alternative to a health club membership? Hey, why not? You're certainly out less money in the long run if in a few months you realize you have neither the time nor inclination for regular exercise. All the same, you won't regret choosing running, both for the cost savings and for the way you're going to feel once you get into it.
- Do you need to fit running into a very busy schedule? If so, you may only have time for a half-hour run a day. That's fine! This book will help you to optimize the time you do have.

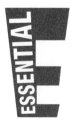
ESSENTIAL

How many times have you intended to change something in your life but it didn't happen? Lots of times, if you're like most people. Well, that's not going to happen this time. You're going to start small, have incremental success, and stay motivated by the growing difference in how you look and feel. You can do this by setting realistic, feel-good goals.

Whatever your short- or long-term goals are for choosing to run, identify them in your notebook so you can be reminded of them. This will keep you focused when the inevitable temptation to do other things comes up. Don't be vague, and decide which is your number one goal, and stick with the program that will get you there. Haphazardly jumping from one training plan to another will only frustrate you and take you further away from achieving something significant. If possible, find a coach and follow her training plan. A qualified coach will consult with you on a regular basis so that your program can be modified should you experience fatigue, soreness, or injury.

Understand the Effects of Running on Your Body

The outlook of this book is that there's no sport like running to help you feel more fit and focused physically and mentally. However, after sharing your new enthusiasm for running you might hear excuses from others that it is bad for your joints, that you are too old, or that running is too time consuming.

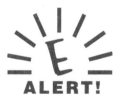
ALERT!

Ask your doctor what she thinks of your starting a running program. You may want to consult a specialist, too, like an orthopedist or someone who handles sports injuries. You may need to prepare your body first before you can start running.

You may not want to listen to this advice, but it's hard not to. Running is a high-impact sport that does affect people's joints differently. Before you incorporate a running program into, say, the countdown for your wedding because you're convinced it's the only way you'll look and feel great—and keep your sanity—in preparation for the big day, be smart and get a physical exam. The last thing you need is an injury if it turns out that you're not biomechanically cut out for this activity. (Chapter 4 provides information on the mechanics of running.)

Choosing and Sticking with a Running Program

Once you are sure of your primary goal and your doctor has given you a green light, you are ready to choose a running program. Not knowing how to start is often the most significant roadblock keeping people from beginning a running program. With the right map in hand, however, you can get started, know where you are going, and enjoy the trip. The following steps will set you up for success.

Schedule Running in Your Life

Pull out your daily planner or calendar and look at the week ahead of you. Schedule your exercise session to fit into your busy schedule. Find a desirable time of day or evening to exercise, and make it a regular habit.

Arrange for family cooperation, if necessary. Perhaps your spouse can trade early morning responsibilities with you; perhaps your children can learn how to make their own breakfast so you can run before taking them to school. When you use your daily planner with an opportunistic eye, you can reserve a small part of your busy day for your exercise time.

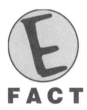

FACT

Although exercising is beneficial at any time of the day, many people prefer running in the morning. This way they have the rest of the day to enjoy the energizing effects of their run.

Think about ways to include family members if they can't be left alone. Buy a baby jogger or stroller and take your youngster with you. Or allow an older child to ride a bike while you run. A child's designated time for homework can be your designated time for body work.

A frequently asked question is: When is the best time of day to do one's body work—morning, afternoon, or evening? The best answer is: The time when you will do it. Some people have a regular schedule that makes it easy for them to plan their exercise at a designated time and day. For others, no two days are alike, and they have to create windows of opportunity for exercise time.

You manage to make time every day for the appointments you can't miss. You get to work on time, pick the kids up from school, go to dentist appointments, and set aside time to read the newspaper or talk on the telephone. You find time for these activities because they are important to you. When you have something important in your life, you are more apt to cherish it and treat it with respect.

Schedule your exercise time as you would other important appointments. Give yourself a start and finish time, and be punctual. A side benefit of setting a regular exercise time is that your partner, boss, children, and coworkers will learn to respect your private exercise time and not to infringe on it unless absolutely necessary.

Make Your Runs Fun and Convenient

Invite a friend, neighbor, or coworker to join you as a regular or even an occasional workout partner. Make sure you choose someone whose company you enjoy so that you will look forward to sharing that time. Ideally, find someone who is also a beginner so that both of you will be running at the same approximate pace.

Canine companions are usually happy to be included on jogs. Make sure that if your dog isn't used to running long distances, you take extra care in conditioning him. You have to remember that his paws and cardiovascular system need time to adapt. And make sure your breed of dog is capable of this type of exercise, of course; you won't get far with a Chihuahua or a Pug, for example.

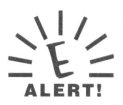

Remember to carry along some water for your canine runner—dogs can overheat quickly. Check out the dog packs that your four-legged friend can carry on his back, remembering to keep the load light. Also, be considerate of how much running your particular dog can handle.

Wear the Right Clothing

Make your runs more enjoyable by investing in workout garb that gives you confidence. Wearing functional and comfortable clothing can make a world of difference in how you feel working out. If you have been saving your worn-out T-shirts, shorts, and sweats for exercise, think again. Those old clothes may not do much for your motivation, especially if you're a beginner who feels a bit self-conscious about running anyway.

There are many useful products available in the marketplace, such as Coolmax and other synthetic-blend fabrics, which are discussed in Chapter 3. These are designed not only to look good but also to help keep you cool, reduce if not eliminate chafing, wick away moisture, and make you feel comfortable.

Start Incrementally and Increase Gradually

When first becoming physically active, more is not always better. Before you learned to walk you had to crawl, and the same is true with your fitness regimen. If you want to be successful with your program and feel good both during and after exercise, you need to start incrementally and then increase time and effort gradually.

This is where many people set themselves up to fail. They expect their body to perform at a level neither realistic nor recommended. Then afterward they wrongly insist the exercise itself made them feel that way. The point here is to be patient and consistent with your exercise plan.

It is particularly important to start slowly if you have not exercised recently. When you first begin to move, it's as if your body has been in a coma. If someone were coming out of a coma, would you shake her and say, "Hey, come on, get going, faster, harder, more, more"? Of course not. Similarly, when you begin an exercise program you should be gentle with your body. If you start slowly, your body will respond favorably. To set yourself up for success, start running for small increments of time at low intensity levels until your body has time to adjust to the new activity. For example, as illustrated in **TABLE 5-1** on page 57, the true beginner might run a total of 2 cumulative minutes in Week Seven, while someone who regularly engages in other types of cardiovascular activities might be able to safely start the program by running 10 consecutive minutes in Week Ten.

Understanding and applying this pacing of fitness will in fact help you to achieve your goal. Some people feel embarrassed by running at a slow pace at first. You need to put this concern aside so you don't set yourself up for injury.

Establish a Foundation

Following the basic principles of exercise establishes a solid foundation for a successful exercise program. These principles are centered around the idea that stressing one's muscles at the appropriate level (the workout) followed by rest leads to the next level of fitness. Understanding this idea can help you determine how to best structure the format of your weekly running schedule. You can optimize your training while increasing your ability at a safe and healthy pace by considering the following factors: frequency (how many days you'll run), intensity (the pace of your runs), time (their duration), and distance (miles). Another factor is the workout type. While the beginner's focus will be to simply run at a relaxed, comfortable pace, the advanced runner can select among a myriad of workout options (hill repeats, intervals, tempo runs, etc. covered in Chapter 11) depending upon her race or fitness goals.

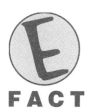

FACT

"After having my second baby, I became frustrated that I had not lost the last 10 pounds of baby weight. This is when I found Art Liberman's mileage buildup program. I dedicated myself to, and completed, the 19-week program. When I finished the 10-mile run, I felt fabulously proud of myself. My self-confidence and self-image soared."—Shelley Barineau, Houston, TX

Fitness expert, author, endurance athlete, and exercise physiologist Sally Edwards states in her book, *Smart Heart*, "You can only manage what you can measure and monitor." This is certainly true for exercise and health. In order to take an active role in your fitness, keep track in your running notebook of what you do, how much you do, and any other relevant information that relates to your health. Be as descriptive as you like. You do not have to be obsessive about every detail but should include enough to tell a story about your exercise and health.

The following is an overview of what you need to get started with your running program to train safely and successfully. These topics are explored in depth later in the book, but they're mentioned briefly here as essential matters to take into consideration when first getting started.

Equipment and Training Log

Buy a new pair of running shoes from someone knowledgeable. The sales staff in specialty running stores are usually runners themselves. They should have the technical knowledge to put you in the right shoes to meet your biomechanical needs. Don't be afraid to ask questions.

When the mileage total of your shoes reaches a maximum of 400 miles, it's time to buy a new pair. You may think 400 miles sounds like a lot, but as you become a more experienced runner mileage total will accrue quickly. Training in shoes that have exceeded their lifespan can lead to a variety of overuse injuries that may take days or even weeks to heal properly. When considering clothing (such as socks, shirts, and shorts), choose those manufactured with synthetic blends that wick away perspiration and reduce the possibility of chafing.

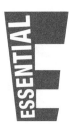

A training log may not seem like an essential item in your quest for fitness, but it is. It's a place to set goals, track achievements, and note ups or downs. You'll be thrilled to look back at the mileage you've run, and in turn you'll be more motivated to stick to your plan.

Another item that will improve your running experience is a training log. Use a notebook, calendar, or running log to record the following information at a minimum: miles run, total time run, and shoe model worn. Some runners record everything from the weather conditions to the route they have run to the total shoe mileage.

Keeping a log is important because it provides a history of your running, which is crucial for finding the possible cause of a running injury. Additionally, reviewing a running log helps to determine the training method that has been most effective in turning out one's best performances. Finally, keeping a log is highly motivating, for few runners like to leave too many blank entries. However, do not become compulsive about your running just to fill in the blanks or reach a specific weekly mileage total come what may.

There are a variety of Web sites that provide training logs and show you how to record everything pertaining to your training program, from actual miles run to cumulative shoe mileage. Best of all, most of these sites are free. (See Appendix C.)

Build a Base

Without question, the most important area to focus on when beginning a running program is that of safely building a mileage base, or the distance you run per week. It's essential to start out running in small increments and build on these, no matter how silly or short your distance seems. Never try to take on too much too soon. Doing so can greatly increase your chances of incurring an overuse injury and may ruin your appetite for running.

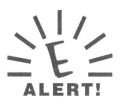

ALERT!

You shouldn't even think of training for a marathon (26.2 miles) until meeting certain conditions. Specifically, you should have been running consistently four to five days per week, 25 miles per week, for at least a year (without any major injuries).

In a chapter on motivation and success, it's hard not to feel like you can strap on your running shoes and do 5 miles easily. Although it's admirable to want to seize the day, remember, slow and steady wins the race. You'll be running an easy 5 miles soon enough if you train smart.

In building your mileage base, remember the 10 percent rule: Do not increase either your weekly mileage and/or your long-run mileage by more than 10 percent a week. Doing so greatly increases the chance of incurring an injury, thereby delaying or stopping your training altogether. This is one of the biggest mistakes runners make. Don't do it!

Without a doubt, runners should include supplemental activities such as weight training and cross-training as part of their total fitness program. In particular, incorporating weight training, stretching, and carefully selected cross-training activities in your fitness regimen both reduces the risk of injury and facilitates total-body conditioning. (You can read more about weight training and cross-training in Chapter 8.)

Nutrition

Nutrition is an essential part of any exercise program. (It is covered in greater detail in Chapter 16.) One thing to keep in mind at this point, though, is that nutrition is not just about food; it's about fluids, too. Runners must be well-hydrated to run effectively. For runs of up to 60 minutes, water is the drink of choice.

It is also important to emphasize healthy foods in your diet and limit fried and high-fat foods. There is much debate now regarding the proper mix of carbohydrates, proteins, and fats. As a runner, you should focus on carbohydrate sources in your diet, aiming for carbohydrates to make up approximately 65 percent of your total daily calories. Split the remaining 35 percent of calories between proteins and fats.

Common Mistakes

Again, making simple, unintentional mistakes is the most common way for runners to derail their programs. Such runners can be categorized into two major groups. The first type adopts the philosophy that "more is better" and builds his mileage too rapidly, thus suffering breakdown and/or injury.

Individuals in the second group are very inconsistent in their training and may miss several workouts in a row. Then, recognizing that they are behind in their training, they'll add on additional miles in an effort to catch up. Neither approach will help you to become a successful runner.

Avoiding Injury

One of the greatest challenges of running is to remain injury free. Although some runners may wear their injuries like a badge of honor, more injuries come from not properly training than from getting hurt on the course. Just as there are different types of runners, there are many types of injuries and treatments.

If you suspect you may have an injury, begin a preventive rehabilitation program to keep the damage to a minimum. Depending on the type of injury, this might mean using ice, over-the-counter anti-inflammatory medication, and above all, resting for a day or two to allow the injury to heal. (Chapter 13 discusses specific ways to greatly reduce your chances of incurring an injury.) Should you experience a minor injury while running, apply RICE. No, not the grain, the principle:

- R = Rest
- I = Ice
- C = Compress
- E = Elevation

If there's swelling or pain, take an anti-inflammatory, such as aspirin or ibuprofen. If your injury doesn't respond to self-treatment in a couple of days, see a doctor.

Stretch Regularly

Beginning runners often underestimate the value of stretching. Stretching is one of the most effective means of avoiding injury and increasing performance and stamina. However, don't stretch a cold muscle before you exercise. It's much safer to stretch after your workout. If a person really wants to stretch beforehand, she should do some brisk walking or a slow 10-minute jog and then stretch. The necessity and benefit of stretching regularly as part of your workout routine cannot be overemphasized.

Utilize Recovery Techniques

There are several therapeutic measures you can take to recover from stressful workouts or from the cumulative effects of hard training over a long period of time. Massage therapy, for example, feels great after a long run, hard race, and/or weeks of heavy training. Another therapeutic technique is pouring cold water on fatigued legs after a race or long workout. You can also try soaking your legs in a whirlpool of warm water (approximately 105°F) a couple of hours after working out. Something as simple as taking a walk or going for an easy bike ride a couple of hours after a hard workout can also work wonders for tired legs.

Chapter 3

The Well-Equipped Runner

Running is one of the least equipment-intensive sports you can participate in. In fact, all you really need to run are shorts, a shirt, and shoes. But if you're going to do it right, you need to know that not just any shorts, shirts, or shoes will do. Appropriate gear should be comfortable and assist you in staying injury free. You can have the trendiest gear money can buy, but if you don't use any of it, so what? Don't get so focused on how you look that you forget that your equipment has to be practical. It has to be easy to care for, easy to take on and off, easy to wash, durable, and comfortable.

Running Shoes

First, you need to outfit your feet with running shoes. These should not be just any running shoes; they should be running shoes that meet your particular biomechanical needs. Take advantage of the fact that running shoes are designed to minimize injury and maximize form and function.

There are three factors to consider in determining the best type of shoe for a particular runner. The first involves what foot type the runner has (high arch, flat foot, or normal arch). It's also important to analyze the runner's footstrike (heel striker, forefoot striker, or midfoot striker) and stride pattern (pronater, supinater, or neutral). (Footstrike and stride pattern will be discussed in detail in Chapter 4.)

Buying the Right Shoes

To be sure that all of these considerations are met when buying your shoes, you should purchase them at a specialty running store rather than at a wholesale sporting goods store. Specialty running stores are places that cater to the needs of runners. Often owned by runners themselves, these stores employ knowledgeable individuals who understand shoe construction and are familiar with the latest models and brands on the market. In short, the staff of specialty running stores are experts in matching your particular foot type and stride pattern to the specific shoe that will best meet your biomechanical needs.

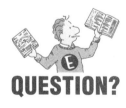

QUESTION?

Is there a best time of the day to try on running shoes?
To get the best and most comfortable fit for your feet, shop later in the day when your feet have swelled to their maximum size. It is also important to remember that there may be several models of running shoes among various brand names (Nike, Saucony, New Balance, Brooks, etc.) that will meet your biomechanical needs. In other words, don't assume that only one brand will work for you.

When being fit for running shoes, try them on with the style of sock (or one of similar thickness) that you will wear when running. When standing in the shoes, you should have a distance equal to the width of your thumb between your longest toe and the end of the shoe. Improperly fitting shoes without enough room between your longest toe and the front of the toebox can lead to black toenails or toenails that fall off. Additionally, your heels should not slip out of the back of the shoes when you walk or run in them.

Since you will be doing more than standing in your running shoes, you will want to run around in them before making your purchase. If the store has space, run around inside, getting off the carpet and onto a hard surface. However, don't run outside with them unless you've asked permission first. If the store won't let you run in them, make sure it has a good return policy. Otherwise, shop at another store.

Types of Running Shoes

Most beginners, as well as people of average to heavy weight, need shoes that provide support, cushioning, and shock absorption. The lighter training shoes (lighter in weight than most running shoes, that is) are designed for experienced runners, for their fast-paced workouts and races. Some lighter-weight runners can also use these shoes. Because they weigh less than most running shoes, they can help shave a few seconds off one's pace. However, due to their lighter weight, they don't offer quite the same degree of protection as a traditional training shoe.

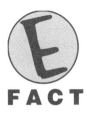

FACT

Because the selection can feel overwhelming (even with the assistance of the knowledgeable staff of a specialty running store), it can be helpful to review shoes online, paying particular attention to user reviews. Search at random, or go to the *Runner's World* magazine Web site (*www .runnersworld.com*).

Racing flats are similar to light-weight trainers but are even lighter in weight and thus offer less protection. Only the advanced competitor should use them for fast-paced, short-distance training sessions and for shorter races.

When selecting a shoe, remember also that shoe companies work hard to get your attention. Their designs and colors are meant to attract you so that you will buy their shoes. However, resist buying a particular style of running shoe because you want to make a fashion statement. You will do yourself a big favor if you think about function over fashion.

The Inside Outs of a Running Shoe

Often when shopping for footwear, you will hear a salesperson use high-tech words to describe the particular features and parts of the running shoe. With a little basic knowledge of running shoes, you can become a more informed buyer and satisfied user. This shoe anatomy session can help you buy the shoe that's right for you.

The toebox refers to the toe section of the shoe. It should be roomy enough to comfortably fit your toes. There should be approximately half an inch between your longest toe and the end of the shoe, and half an inch between the top of your longest toe and the top of the toebox.

Next, take a look at shoe laces. You should use laces that are not too long or too slippery. If they are too long, cut them down or use lace locks.

Held together by the laces is the upper, or the material that encloses the foot. Breathable fabrics such as mesh keep feet from overheating in the summer. When choosing a shoe, be sure the upper fits properly; it helps the shoe stabilize the foot.

Beneath the laces you will find the tongue of the shoe. The tongue should be thick enough to protect the top of the foot from the pressure of the laces, but not so long that it rubs against your foot just above the ankle.

At the back of the shoe is the heel notch, the slight depression cut into the shoe's heel collar to reduce Achilles tendon irritation and provide a more secure heel fit. The heel counter is the rounded place where your heel fits snugly yet comfortably. Too loose a fit can cause blisters on your heels. If you need extra stability (for instance, your feet wobble a lot), look for a stiff heel counter or an external heel counter (a ring that wraps around the outside of the heel). On the bottom of the shoe, look for the split heel, a two-part heel structure that separates the outer and inner sides and contributes to a smoother heel-to-toe transition.

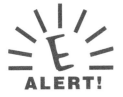

ALERT!

Occasionally, runners complain about their feet feeling tingly or numb, particularly during longer training runs. This is sometimes attributed to shoelaces being tied too tightly, which reduces the circulation of blood to one's feet. A simple solution for this annoying problem is to tie your laces just tightly enough that your shoes stay snugly on your feet.

Look for heel heights that match your cushioning needs. If you are a big person, chances are you are more of a heel-striker and want more midsole foam under the heel, so you need a greater heel height. Faster runners tend to strike more in the midfoot and need a lower heel.

Getting to Know Your Soles

Most of the cushioning and shock absorption in shoes is provided by the midsole, the part of the shoe that you can't see (located above the outer sole). You will want one of two midsole foams: polyurethane or eva. Polyurethane is denser, heavier, and more durable than eva. Eva is a softer, cushier material. Generally, heavier runners do well with polyurethane midsoles. Eva is more common because of its lightness and more cushioned feel.

The material that covers the bottom of the shoe is referred to as the outer sole. You will want one of three kinds of outer sole: carbon rubber, blown rubber, or a combination of the two. Carbon rubber is more durable, but heavier and stiffer, than blown rubber. Some shoes have carbon rubber in the high-wear areas of the rear foot and the cushier blown rubber in the forefoot for a softer feel.

Running shoes also contain stabilizing technology, or devices that reduce overpronation. These are usually in the shoe's midsole on the arch side of the shoe. Some shoes have firmer densities of midsole foam to combat overpronation. (Pronation and overpronation will be discussed in greater detail in Chapter 4.)

Wearing and Caring for Your Running Shoes

One important aspect to consider in wearing running shoes is how you lace them. Lacing your shoes may sound like a silly thing to discuss, but how you do it can make a tremendous difference in how your feet feel in the shoes. Does your heel slip in your shoes? Does the top of your foot get irritated or fall asleep? If so, the following lacing remedies should help you.

For heel slippage, if your heel moves side to side or up and down, try using the shoe's lace lock. This will bring the heel of the shoe closer to your heel, alleviating the slipping.

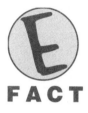

FACT

Lace locking to prevent heel slippage is something you can do with any pair of lace-up shoes. To do it, lace normally from the bottom all the way to the next-to-last eyelet. When you bring the lace out of that eyelet, instead of crossing over to the other one, go straight up to the top eyelet and bring the lace through to the back. Do this on both sides of the shoe. Bring the excess lace across and through the small tab you now have at the very top of the shoe, then tie your shoe. This will give you a tight fit at the ankle but not over the rest of your foot.

If the top of your foot falls asleep or gets irritated, you may have a high instep. A high instep causes your foot to take up an excessive amount of space in your shoe. However, if your foot slides around in your shoe and tightening your laces doesn't fix the problem, you may have a narrow foot. In this case, purchase shoes from manufacturers that offer width-sizing options.

Take care of your running shoes, and they will take care of you. It's very important to make sure you keep your shoes in the best possible condition. Worn-out shoes can lead to unwelcome aches and pains or even injury. Follow these tips, and your feet and legs will thank you for it:

- Wear your running shoes only for running—they will last much longer.
- If your shoes become dirty, hand wash them with commercial shoe care products rather than machine washing and drying them.

- When your running shoes become wet, stick crumpled-up newspaper inside them to accelerate the drying time.

Adding Orthotics

When you think about it, since every foot is unique, it's amazing that shoes that fit well and support your movements can be mass-produced to satisfy so many. The truth is, though, that only about one person in four has a normal running pattern. The rest have feet that either turn too much or not enough when their heels hit the ground. Shoe manufacturers cater to over- and underpronators (learn more about pronation in Chapter 4), but such runners are still more susceptible to injury.

It wasn't too long ago that if you suffered a foot-related injury you had to go to a sports podiatrist and have a pair of prescription orthotics custom-made for your feet. Not always an insurance-covered expense, orthotics could cost several hundred dollars. Though definitely worth it for those passionate about running, this solution could be potentially discouraging or even a last straw for those struggling with the sport.

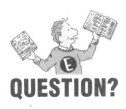

QUESTION?

What is an orthotic?
An orthotic is a piece of specially designed, molded material that is inserted into shoes to compensate for the wearer's biomechanical inefficiencies.

Today runners can try reducing injury as a result of their imperfect strides by supplementing their running shoes with over-the-counter orthotics. Certainly superior to foam-cushioned insoles, these inserts are designed to provide maximum shock absorption while compensating for pronation and other irregularities. It's important to speak with someone knowledgeable about biomechanics and running shoes before simply ditching the sock liner of your new shoes and putting in an otc orthotic you think will help. In fact, without proper understanding of its purpose, your use of an orthotic may increase your risk of injury.

Running Socks

Some people tend to take socks for granted, but it only takes one blister to bring your feet to your attention. A general rule in choosing socks is that activities that produce a lot of foot friction require a thicker sock. For example, sports like basketball and racquetball generate a lot of friction and warrant thicker socks. Unless you are running on trails (which can create high friction), you can be comfortable running in a thin sock, but again, go with what feels good to you.

There are numerous synthetic fabrics being used today that make socks fit, hold up, and wick away moisture better than ever before (so that you don't have wet feet, which can cause blisters). There is also no need to suffer with socks that bunch and slip down into your shoes. These will only irritate you while running and may produce some nasty blisters.

The Right Fit

The fit of your socks can make a tremendous difference in your exercise comfort. Your socks should not constrict your skin nor make a deep imprint upon it, especially at the ankles or calves. Socks are meant to support the foot, reduce friction, regulate foot temperature, and promote comfort and circulation, not restrict it. Your socks should not bunch up inside your shoes or slide off your feet, and you should be able to move your feet and wiggle your toes comfortably. Whether you're running simply for overall fitness or to complete a marathon, you can help ensure a pain-free running experience by experimenting with a variety of sock styles until you find the type that best works for you.

Additional Support Wear

In addition to shoes and socks, you may be in need of additional support wear for your body. Running creates a lot of movement and vibration of the body that can cause discomfort. Fortunately, there are many products on the market to aid both men and women in exercise comfort.

Athletic Supporters, Jock Straps, and Compression Shorts

Personal preference dictates the use of these invaluable protective and supportive devices for boys and men. For contact activities (martial arts) and even some nonintentional contact sports (soccer), athletic cups and supporters may be preferred. Neither of these is really necessary for running. However, support for men is still a big issue. Two garment styles that have taken the place of more traditional supporters are running shorts with built-in liners and compression shorts. They reduce movement and vibration, which leads to greater comfort.

Sports Bras

Unlike male support mechanisms that have been around a long time, sports bras were first introduced in the late 1970s. They didn't become widely accepted until the 1980s, when the real running boom hit.

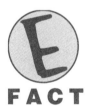

FACT

In July 1999, American soccer player Brandi Chastain's winning penalty kick gave her team the World Cup championship. Chastain, in pure joy, spontaneously pulled off her jersey, revealing her sports bra. At that moment, the sports bra took center stage like never before. Chastain's moment of celebration was captured on the cover of *Newsweek* with the caption "Girls Rule!"

There are three types of sports bras: compression, encapsulation, and combination. Compression-style bras use the pressure of the fabric to squeeze or press the breasts flat against the chest, limiting movement. Small- to medium-breasted women favor this style. The encapsulation style limits movement by surrounding and supporting the breasts with reinforced seams or wire (like an underwire bra). Larger-breasted women prefer this style. The combination style combines compression and encapsulation.

There are many options for sports bras, and women are all healthier and happier for them. Comfort should ultimately dictate a woman's choice. The options include underwire, wireless, rear clasp, front clasp, no clasp, front zipper, cross-over-the-head, cross-in-the-back, cross-in-the-front, halter style, nursing compatible, prosthetic compatible, heart rate monitor encapsulated, high impact, and low impact. Most of these bras also come in a variety of great colors and styles.

Other Running Necessities

Depending on the weather and how comfortable you'll be wearing them, you might want to run with one or more of the following: sunglasses, a sweatband, a baseball cap, a wool hat, gloves, and a key and/or change carrier that can be wrapped around your wrist, ankle, or waist. You can get as low-tech or high-tech as you want, now that there are materials that reflect or absorb light, wick moisture away from your skin, insulate while remaining lightweight and dry, and so on. If you run at night, you'll need reflective gear (or you can sew or glue reflective tape to your gear). Also, don't forget sunscreen when you're out during the day. You'll need it in the winter as much as in the summer.

A Running Watch

You will come to depend on your running watch the way you depend on your wristwatch when you think you might be late for work. Your running watch will let you know how you're doing at all times.

The watch you use doesn't have to be expensive (though it can be). Before purchasing a watch for running, decide what functions you think you'll really use. Most include a stopwatch, an alarm, lap settings (also called split timing), a glow light for seeing your time at night, and a regular watch. Make sure the model you choose isn't too complicated or intimidating. The stopwatch will be the part you use most, so make sure it's easy to start, stop, and reset, and is also waterproof.

But why simply monitor your overall time and distance when you can learn so much more about your performance during a run? There are a variety of models that enable you to continuously monitor your speed, distance, pace, calories burned, and heart rate throughout the various phases of your workout. You can even make your workouts more challenging with a virtual partner feature, enabling you to train alongside a digital competitor with programmable specified time, distance, and pace goals. Some devices feature the capability of downloading information to a computer so you can both store the data and keep an online running log.

Water, Water Anywhere

Although a runner's best friend in the short run is water, workouts longer than 60 minutes additionally require a consumption of sports drinks—critical both for keeping heat-driven illness at bay as well as for ensuring optimal performance. Organized races set up aid stations to be sure runners stay hydrated. In the old days when going it alone, there were limited options for staying hydrated. Carrying a water bottle in your hand can compromise your running form and is awkward as the water sloshes and gets warm. Before setting out, you might fill your stomach to the limit, risking a need to relieve yourself in midrun (or worse, underestimating the quantity of fluids needed for the weather conditions or distance and not consuming nearly enough fluids). An effective but time-consuming option is to plan your route and stash water and sports drink bottles along the way. Thankfully, today there are now practical and convenient carrying systems available that you can strap onto your waist and that hold a variety of plastic bottle sizes. Other systems strap to your back and include fluid delivery tubes, making sipping easy and convenient so you can access water at all times.

Jog to the Music

Some runners consider the gear they use to listen to music while they run as important as their clothes, watch, or even fluids. With portable music systems getting increasingly smaller and lighter, it is infinitely easier and more comfortable to get into the groove with your favorite selection of Motown, funk, classic rock, classical music, or even talk radio than ever before. Runners compare and contrast play lists on their iPods as frequently as they do split-times or which races are their favorites. Like chatting with a running buddy, listening to music can make a run feel less challenging and shorter—and who doesn't appreciate that? Runners who use portable music-playing systems need to be especially mindful of their surroundings, however.

The Runner's Log

How does a training log qualify as equipment? Because without it, you're running in the dark. As discussed in Chapter 2, there are three main reasons for keeping a log. First, the log provides a history of your running, crucial to finding a possible cause of a running injury. Second, reviewing a running log helps determine which training methods have been most effective in prompting one's best performances. Finally, keeping a log is highly motivating, since few runners like to leave too many empty lines. (See **TABLE 3-1** for an example log.) Additionally, it's useful to keep a shoe mileage chart (see **TABLE 3-2**), which makes it easy to determine when it's time to purchase a new pair of shoes (when your shoes reach an upper limit of 400 miles).

What to Log

At a minimum, you need to record the distance you have actually covered in your workout. This total should also include your warm-up and cool-down mileage because, after all, you did cover that distance on foot.

You should estimate your average pace per mile running by time rather than by mileage. To do this, you can visit a track and run 4 laps at a relaxed pace (four times around most high school or college tracks equals 1,600 meters, or very close to a mile). Then run for a specific amount of time and determine the mileage covered. For example, if your easy pace for a mile is 9 minutes, run for a little over 36 minutes, and call the workout a 4-miler.

The next item to log is the time duration of your workout. In other words, determine how many total minutes you were moving and running, walking, or a combination of both. If you are using the walk/run method of training, you can be even more specific if you like by recording the actual minutes you were running and the minutes you were walking.

Table 3-1
Runner's Log

Week of:		Sun.	Mon.	Tues.	Wed.	Thurs.	Fri.	Sat.	Total
__/__ to __/__	Time								
	Mileage								
__/__ to __/__	Time								
	Mileage								
__/__ to __/__	Time								
	Mileage								
__/__ to __/__	Time								
	Mileage								
__/__ to __/__	Time								
	Mileage								
__/__ to __/__	Time								
__/__ to __/__	Mileage								
	Time								
__/__ to __/__	Mileage								
	Time								
__/__ to __/__	Mileage								
	Time								
__/__ to __/__	Mileage								
	Time								

Table 3-2
Shoe Mileage Chart

Pair #1_____			Pair #2_____			Pair #3_____		
Date	D.M.	C.M.	Date	D.M.	C.M.	Date	D.M.	C.M.
Date	D.M.	C.M.	Date	D.M.	C.M.	Date	D.M.	C.M.
Date	D.M.	C.M.	Date	D.M.	C.M.	Date	D.M.	C.M.
Date	D.M.	C.M.	Date	D.M.	C.M.	Date	D.M.	C.M.
Date	D.M.	C.M.	Date	D.M.	C.M.	Date	D.M.	C.M.
Date	D.M.	C.M.	Date	D.M.	C.M.	Date	D.M.	C.M.
Date	D.M.	C.M.	Date	D.M.	C.M.	Date	D.M.	C.M.
Date	D.M.	C.M.	Date	D.M.	C.M.	Date	D.M.	C.M.
Date	D.M.	C.M.	Date	D.M.	C.M.	Date	D.M.	C.M.
Date	D.M.	C.M.	Date	D.M.	C.M.	Date	D.M.	C.M.
Date	D.M.	C.M.	Date	D.M.	C.M.	Date	D.M.	C.M.
Date	D.M.	C.M.	Date	D.M.	C.M.	Date	D.M.	C.M.
Date	D.M.	C.M.	Date	D.M.	C.M.	Date	D.M.	C.M.
Date	D.M.	C.M.	Date	D.M.	C.M.	Date	D.M.	C.M.
Date	D.M.	C.M.	Date	D.M.	C.M.	Date	D.M.	C.M.
Date	D.M.	C.M.	Date	D.M.	C.M.	Date	D.M.	C.M.
Date	D.M.	C.M.	Date	D.M.	C.M.	Date	D.M.	C.M.
Date	D.M.	C.M.	Date	D.M.	C.M.	Date	D.M.	C.M.
Date	D.M.	C.M.	Date	D.M.	C.M.	Date	D.M.	C.M.
Date	D.M.	C.M.	Date	D.M.	C.M.	Date	D.M.	C.M.
Date	D.M.	C.M.	Date	D.M.	C.M.	Date	D.M.	C.M.
Date	D.M.	C.M.	Date	D.M.	C.M.	Date	D.M.	C.M.
Date	D.M.	C.M.	Date	D.M.	C.M.	Date	D.M.	C.M.

Key: D.M. = Daily Mileage; C.M. = Cumulative Mileage

For runners who rotate two or more pairs of running shoes for their training from day to day, or even if you own just one pair, it's also important to write down the shoe model you used for your workout and the respective miles run in that particular shoe. This will enable you to track its wear. Many injuries can be traced to training shoes that are worn out.

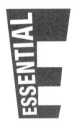

To log your information, you can use a blank calendar or a spiral notebook. *Runner's World* also puts out a comprehensive training log that you can use to record your workouts for an entire year. There are also a variety of free Web sites that enable you to record the specifics of your workout (mileage, shoes, duration, etc.). In short, the choice is yours.

Other indicators you can record include, but are not limited to, heart rate (for those runners who use a monitor before and during exercise), weather (temperature, wind, conditions), the specific route you ran, how your legs felt during and after the workout, other cross-training activities done that day, what you had to eat, how much water you took in, and so on. The key is to have a program of what you are willing to record on a day-by-day basis.

Using a Calendar

Another way to keep a log is by using a calendar. This can sometimes be better than a separate log because you can also use it to record other events in your life. This gives you an understanding of how other events can be distractions or hindrances to your running. One drawback to calendars is that they are not always easy to write on and don't offer the space to write more extensive notations. Even so, calendars are easy to maintain and give you the opportunity to make running part of your everyday life.

Chapter 4

The Mechanics of Running

Is there really a right way to run? Conversely, is there a wrong way to run? The answer to both questions is yes. However, that does not mean that everyone should run in the same way with the same form. The fact is that form varies from runner to runner. Every person's form emerges naturally over time. The objective of this chapter is to teach you about form and what happens when you run so that you can maximize your natural running efficiencies and minimize what can lead to injury.

4

Assessing Running Form

Many of the fastest runners are not necessarily naturally gifted; neither are they by necessity exceptionally tall or long limbed. Instead, the best runners are those with economical strides and who run with purpose, power, and determination. Not only can good form make the difference between running pain free and running with pain, but good form can also shave minutes off your running time.

Improving one's speed poses the greatest challenge for a runner. Many runners (both beginners and intermediates) lean forward and run on their toes to try to go faster. This is a sprinting technique. Trying to run a 5K or 10K in this manner will probably result in pain and may even lead to injury. Additionally, running in this way can hinder a runner from achieving her fastest possible pace.

Speed can also be affected by bouncing. Bouncing slows the runner down and is extremely inefficient. It creates greater impact on the legs, especially the knees. Bouncers tend not to pick their knees up very high, and sometimes swing their legs in an excessive and inefficient manner, possibly leading to pain or injury.

There are other problems regarding form that plague runners. Many of these problems are not readily recognizable. However, once recognized, they are easily corrected. Although you don't have to have perfect form, even a minor adjustment or modification can make a tremendous difference in your running efficiency and comfort level. Additionally, tweaking your form a bit can reduce your chances of incurring an injury.

The next time you go to a 5K road race or a popular running trail, you should stop and check out the other runners. You can tell good form from improper or inefficient form just by watching. How? The runners with good form appear more graceful; they have an economy of movement and a certain style that seems natural and easy while incorporating good mechanics.

While watching them, take note of what they are doing. Is their forward motion smoother than yours? Are they carrying their arms lower than you? Are they running less on their toes? Are they running with better posture? Observing and contemplating how to improve your overall mechanics is an excellent way to learn.

Style and Mechanics

Your running style refers to how you run. Beginning runners should try running as naturally as possible while keeping in mind the proper mechanics (explained below). Knowing and maintaining these mechanics leads to more efficient form. Don't push yourself to run fast right away. That is how many beginning runners burn out. Instead, concentrate first on comfort and form. The way to approach running as a new way of life is first to learn the right habits and then perfect them. After you've been running for a few months, it's a good idea to ask an experienced runner or (preferably) a coach to point out and correct your form flaws or deficiencies. This, in turn, will improve your overall mechanics and running efficiency.

Principles to keep in mind when you run:

- **Run relaxed.** Tension saps energy and causes fatigue to set in earlier.
- **Run naturally.** Develop your own running style, all the while employing good running techniques and mechanics.
- **Run tall.** Good posture while you run creates other good habits like knee lift, natural extension of stride, and better breathing.

Mechanics are the individual functions of the body during running. The main mechanics include: breathing; footstrike, also referred to as footprint; stride; arms and hands, or armstride; and posture. Each of these areas can affect your efficiency, your comfort, and your results.

Although you cannot change completely the way in which you run and you cannot change your bone and muscle structure, you can make an effort to become a smoother, more efficient runner by correcting any bad habits you have unknowingly developed. By knowing the basics of good mechanics, you can improve your running form.

Breathing

One of the most vital yet underrated areas you can work on to improve your running efficiency is correct breathing technique. The problem is that many people breathe from their chest rather than from their abdominal region while they run.

Even chest breathers with good lungs may have some trouble breathing while running. Don't worry if you're making too much noise with your breathing while running. You may wheeze, snort, cough, or grunt. As long as you're not overexerting yourself, these noises are harmless.

Whether you're a beginner or an experienced runner, take the time to learn and employ the abdominal breathing method. At a minimum, just remember to keep breathing deeply and regularly. In most cases your breathing will take care of itself; as you run faster, you'll breathe faster. And yes, most runners are mouth breathers or at least nose and mouth breathers. It would be impossible to take in adequate oxygen just breathing through your nose.

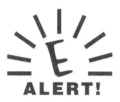

ALERT!

A secret to breathing better when you run is to remember to put a little more force into your exhalation. Your body will naturally inhale to make up for this, which in turn will improve your breathing efficiency.

Establishing Your Breathing Rhythm

Your breathing rhythm is very important. Rhythm and stride are closely related to your breathing, so make breathing a top priority as you progress through your training program. Whether you take three strides for every breath or two, your breathing and your stride are probably in sync naturally. Beginning runners, though, make the mistake of breathing at a 1:1 rate. This means that they are taking one step while breathing in and one step while breathing out. This is essentially panting, and it is inefficient breathing.

The more economical way to breathe depends, to a large degree, on the pace at which you are running. For your average run, you should breathe 2:2

(taking two steps for every breath in and two steps for every breath out) or 3:3 for longer, slower runs. As you run faster, you may have to breathe more often, which leads to such variations as 2:1 and 1:2 patterns.

All about Footstrike

Footstrike, or footprint, is how your foot strikes the ground. The footprint is what you leave behind. Each footstrike is like your signature as a runner. Do you run on your toes? Do you run heel to toe? Do you run flat footed? The way your foot comes into contact with the ground is very important. Although you probably cannot change your footstrike significantly, making minor adjustments to correct faulty foot mechanics enables you to run more efficiently. These corrections include being fitted for the proper shoe to match your biomechanical needs or adding an orthotic or arch support to your shoe. (Chapter 3 discusses shoe selection and orthotics in greater detail.)

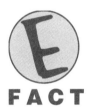

FACT

Studies have shown that short- and middle-distance runners first strike the ground with the ball of the foot rather than midfoot or between midfoot and heel. Beginning and intermediate runners should use the heel-ball footstrike (described on pages 46–47), as it allows for better shock absorption, less stress on the calf muscle and Achilles tendon, and better rolling and push off to the next stride.

Footstrike Types

There are three basic types of footstrikes: normal/neutral, overpronated, and supinated (also called underpronated). In the normal, or neutral, footstrike, the foot rolls slightly inward as it strikes. Your foot flattens out as it makes full contact with the ground, then rolls inward to the center of the body. This inward roll of your foot while running, called pronation, is actually a good thing, since it absorbs some of the force placed on the foot during the normal exercise of running.

Only about 25 percent of the population pronates normally, however, leaving the rest to figure out how to compensate. Overpronation occurs when contact with the ground is first made through the outside of the heel. This causes the foot to roll excessively inward upon contact and the push to come from the big toe and second toe. Overpronation is oftentimes seen in those who have flat feet. Running-shoe models designed and constructed with motion control or stability features help reduce the degree of overpronation. This in turn helps prevent a wide array of overuse injuries that can occur if overpronation is left unchecked.

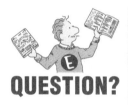

QUESTION?

Which footstrike are you?
Give yourself a footprint test to determine this. While barefoot, put a piece of cardboard on the floor, wet the bottom of your foot, and press firmly and with a solid walking motion on the cardboard to leave an impression of the bottom of your foot in motion. If your footprint appears flat and shows almost your entire foot, you are probably an overpronator. If your footprint shows little or no connecting band between your heel and the ball of your foot, you probably have high arches and are an underpronator.

Supination, or underpronation, also occurs when the outside of the heel makes initial contact. In this instance, however, the foot doesn't roll inward enough upon hitting the ground, resulting in the outside of the foot taking too much of the impact and push off being done by the smaller toes. Characteristic of runners with high arches, supination minimizes the ability of the foot—and, in turn, the legs—to absorb shock, which can lead to injury. To counteract supination, runners with this type of footstrike should wear running shoes that are well-cushioned and flexible. It's extremely important to know whether you are a normal pronator, an overpronator, or a supinator before you buy your running shoes so that you can get a pair that helps you compensate appropriately.

The Toes' Role in Footstrike

Regardless of what kind of footstrike you have, you also need to keep your toes in mind. If not totally awkward for you, try to run with your toes pointed forward. Sometimes, especially when you are tired, your feet don't always point forward when you run. In order to get the most power and efficiency from your push off, work on keeping your feet pointed straight ahead as you run. Doing so results in greater efficiency, which in turn enables you to run faster with the same cardiovascular effort. In short, toes and feet that aren't pointed in the right direction result in wasted and inefficient motion.

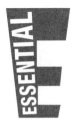

Go for a run paying particular attention to your footstrike. Run naturally and, if possible, past windows in which to see your reflection. This allows you to adjust any flaws in your form or posture, which will make you a more efficient runner.

Of course, this advice is intended for those who need to adjust faulty technique in order to improve their form and thus reduce their chance of injury. Some runners are not put together in a way that allows them to have a "perfect" footfall. For them, a forced effort to run a certain way can actually create a problem worse than poor running form.

Another thing to focus on while running is to try to make sure your toes are the last thing off the ground. This enables you to achieve more power from your stride, resulting in more forward momentum. One's footstrike should be a singular springing motion that is fluid and graceful, resulting in a balanced impact and a powerful push off.

Flat, Heel, and Toe Footstrikes

Many beginners run with a flat footstrike, characterized by landing on a flat foot and having little or no push off. This isn't particularly bad or wrong. If this is the way you run, especially in the beginning, don't change it. Run naturally. To improve your speed and overall efficiency, however, you eventually need to make some adjustments to your footstrike and push off. This is discussed later in this chapter.

Other than a flat footstrike, the heel strike is the most common footstrike of beginning runners. With a heel strike, your heel lands first, then you roll along the outer border of your foot until your midfoot makes contact with the ground. Your toes then make contact with the ground as your heel lifts up, and eventually your foot comes off the ground. If this is how you run, you should not change this, at least not when you first begin a running program. It is a very normal and natural footstrike.

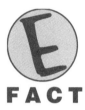

FACT

In an attempt to improve their speed, many beginning runners compensate by employing either the heel or toe footstrike method. Over time, both methods increase the wear and tear on one's legs, so try to avoid them whenever possible.

The heel strike technique is perfectly fine for longer, slower running. However, as with the flat footstrike, to gain the speed and efficiency that shorter runs and races require, you should adopt the midfoot-strike footprint.

Many beginners stomp when they run, hitting too hard with their feet. Your heel should land gently on the ground. If your feet are slapping the ground and making an audible noise even when you're striking with your heel first, you need to make a serious change. Land gently on your heel and roll your foot forward to the midfoot and then the toes, from which you can push off.

Another type of footstrike is the toe strike. This is a footstrike in which only your toes and midfoot make contact with the ground. This is a sprinting technique and is not appropriate for distance running. Therefore, unless you are a sprinter, don't purposely run on your toes.

Heel-Ball and Ball-Heel-Toe Footstrikes

The preferred method of footstrike for the beginner, intermediate, and heavier runner is the heel-ball strike. (For the purpose of this discussion, the ball of your foot is the area that starts at the deep base of your big toe and goes across your foot to your smallest toe.) Although in the heel-ball footstrike the heel strikes first, this is almost simultaneous with the lowering of the ball of the foot. This footstrike allows for minimum impact over a long period of time yet has enough push off to generate speed.

A more advanced footstrike technique is the ball-heel-toe strike, in which you land on the outside edge of the ball of your foot, bring your foot down so your heel touches the ground, and then roll back up to push off with your big toe. This technique is for advanced runners rather than for beginners. Because beginners are still in the process of developing the musculoskeletal components in their legs, they thereby increase their risk of injury by employing this footstrike style. The ball-heel-toe footstrike is appropriate to use when you can average under 7 minutes per mile in a 5K.

It's All about Stride

Stride concerns how your legs swing into position as you run. Some people have long, loping strides, while others have short, economical ones. Some lift their knees high, while others barely lift them at all. Stride can make a huge difference in how well you run. Most runners who want to increase their speed turn to adjusting their stride in order to make it to the next level.

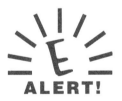

ALERT!

Even though it has always been considered a good thing to have a little bounce in your step, in running circles it is a sign that something is wrong. Don't bounce or bound; it means that you are overstriding. If you shorten your stride and eliminate bouncing, you conserve energy that can be better used to propel yourself forward.

Start with your natural stride, and see where it takes you. Don't be concerned with trying to run fast when you first begin a running program. As beginning runners progress through the first few months of their running program and want to improve their efficiency and speed, there are three adjustments that can be considered: stride frequency, stride length, and knee lift.

Stride Length

Stride length refers to how far you are stepping out when you extend your leg and foot. Increasing your stride length increases the amount of ground you cover with each step. However, make sure not to overextend your stride, since this, too, is inefficient.

A good rule of thumb is for your heel not to strike the ground too far in front of your knee. Some running experts feel that a short stride is a sign of inflexibility. That is not always so. Proper stretching after a run can help to improve your flexibility, which can lengthen your stride.

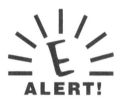
ALERT!

Don't kick your legs up when you run. Some runners kick their heels way up behind them when they run, wasting motion and energy. To get the optimum power from your stride, you should extend your leg behind you when pushing off, then bring it forward as soon as possible.

Overstriders are easy to spot since they usually have an excessive kick or else rarely bend their knees. They tend to lope or bounce, and their motion is not rhythmic or fluid. Overstriding can actually slow you down due to feet being in contact with the ground longer than for a normal stride length. Make sure you don't overstride, as it can lead to a host of problems including Achilles tendonitis, iliotibial band pain, and iliopsoas muscle pain.

Stride Frequency

Increasing the frequency of your stride is a little more challenging than increasing its length. You're asking your body to move faster than it already is, which isn't an easy thing to do. Basically, you are asking your body to quicken its natural rhythm. One way to improve your stride frequency is by concentrating on your knee motion.

Knee Lift

By focusing on your knee motion, you'll probably improve both your stride frequency and length. Be careful not to bring your knees up too high, because how far you bring your knees up determines how long your stride will be. Remember, a stride that's too long or too short is inefficient. Therefore, the correct knee lift coupled with the correct frequency of leg turnover dictates how effectively you can cover ground. In short, the knees do not have to come up very high for long-distance runners. Only sprinters or those charging up a hill have to lift their legs a bit higher than usual.

Arms and Hands

The way you carry your arms helps to provide balance and power while running. Many feel there is a correlation between moving their arms faster and getting their legs to move faster. Optimally, the arms should support the energy of the body in a forward motion while running.

Your arms provide balance in the following way: As your left leg goes forward, so does your right arm. This balances you as you move forward. Then when the right leg moves forward, so does the left arm. How you carry your arms while moving is called arm carriage.

For proper arm carriage, your hands should be shaped in a fist, lightly clasped rather than tightly clinched. Don't waste muscle power needlessly. This isn't a stress test, so relax. Leave your fists slightly open, and as you move allow your arms to swing, carrying them at your side somewhere between your waist and your chest. Make sure they are not too high or too low. One arm swings forward while the other one goes backward in conjunction with the opposite foot and leg motion.

Different types of runners have different types of arm carriage. Sprinters move their arms in a straight forward-backward motion. Most longer-distance runners use a slight arc as they swing their arms, but the faster, more efficient ones don't waste motion by moving too much from side to side. In other words, they don't swing their arms excessively in front of their body.

Wasted motion in the arms is just as bad as an improper or inefficient stride in the legs. A few arm carriage Don'ts include:

- Don't carry your arms too high, which makes your stride shorter than it should be and might result in tightness in your back.
- Don't carry your arms too low, lest your body lean too far forward or in a side-to-side motion due to improper balance.
- Don't swing your elbows out too wide, since this, too, results in throwing your balance off and negatively affecting your stride.
- Don't swing your arms too far inward, as this can increase your chance of incurring hip injuries.

Posture

One of the biggest mistakes beginners make is to employ poor body posture when they run. Unless you're racing the 200 meters (or shorter), don't lean forward. Doing so places great stress on your back and knees.

Proper posture begins with the correct body angle. To get a sense of this body angle, stand up straight against a wall. Your chest should be up but not out, your shoulders relaxed, and your buttocks pushed firmly back. This is the posture in which you should run. It allows for correct breathing, prevents you from leaning over and placing too much stress on your knees, lower legs, and back, and helps you to lengthen your stride and make knee lift easier. It also helps you to have a more efficient footstrike.

In thinking about your posture as you run, you should consider where your hips are when your foot hits the ground. Some people have suggested that your foot when it strikes the ground should be under the center of gravity of your body. A line from your head through your hips should end up at your foot. Keep your head fairly straight and look ahead. Turns to the side should be done carefully and usually mostly from the neck up to avoid twisting your body and making you unstable in your forward progression. You should run standing up fairly straight, not leaning forward, twisted to one side, or tilting backward. Look ahead at where you are going, and don't stare at your feet or at the ground.

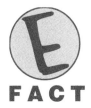

FACT

An Austrian actor named F.M. Alexander, who lost his voice because he was clenching his throat muscles, developed a posture-enhancing technique known today the world over as the Alexander Technique. Beneficial for anyone from daylong computer users to professional athletes, the Alexander Technique, in helping you become more aware of your posture, takes stress off your body and enables you to move more freely.

As you are running, also be careful not to stick your chest out, since doing so increases tightness and tension in all the muscles in your back and neck. Your shoulders should be relaxed. As you're able to build up time and mileage, your back may tighten up sometimes, usually because you're becoming tense. Therefore, even as you focus on good posture, remember to relax. You want to run standing up straight, but comfortably so.

The Mechanics of Running Hills

Because running on level ground requires different mechanics than going up and down hills, what benefits a long-distance runner can fail you in negotiating hills successfully. One of the few good things about hills is that they force you to use muscles you don't normally use.

Running Uphill

Even though you won't be able to maintain the same speed running uphill as you do on the flats, try to maintain the same effort level. Move your arms a bit more to assist your legs. Imagine that you are cranking your way up or pulling yourself up the hill. Shorten your stride, lift your knees a bit, lean slightly into the hill, and power on up.

Running Downhill

One of the best things about running downhill is that you can use gravity to your advantage. However, few people know how to really negotiate the downhill side effectively without losing control or slowing down. Although your natural tendency is to lean back when going downhill, you should instead lean forward slightly to maintain a posture in relation to the ground, as if you were running on the flat. Try to keep your foot-strike light so as not to grind your heels into the hill as a braking mechanism. Use slight upper body positioning to make speed and body balance adjustments.

Runners with little prior experience with downhill running should be careful. The biggest risk of injury is to your knees. Your quadriceps do the bulk of the braking and can be overworked without you being aware of it.

If you are racing in a short race, you may lean forward a bit and fly down the hill, but certainly be more careful in training. In fact, many runners who use hills as part of their advanced training walk or lightly jog down a hill to recover before charging up again. This is a good way to rest and recover while avoiding the excessive knee stress that downhill running can cause.

Runner's Recap

As you develop proper running technique, remember the essentials of running mechanics. First, your posture should be guided by a focus on standing erect, imagining a cord coming out of the center and top of your head that gently pulls you straight up. Use your neck muscles to keep your head looking forward, not buried in your chest nor cocked back. Additionally, as you run, keep your face relaxed by letting your jaw drop and your cheeks flap, and keep your eyes looking about 10–20 feet ahead of you.

Concentrating on your body while running, pull up with your abdominal muscles, and focus on running tall with your torso perpendicular to the running surface and your hips directly under your upper body. Let your shoulders hang relaxed and low, not drawn up toward your ears. Hold your arms close to your body, bending them at ninety-degree angles and keeping them near parallel to the ground as they swing counter to your legs. At the same time, hold your hands in a loose fist, with your thumbs up and your palms facing each other.

With a light, efficient, short stride, each foot should land directly under the center of your body weight, not out in front of you. You should land lightly on your heel or ball (midfoot), roll forward onto the ball of your foot, then push off with the balls of your feet and toes in a smooth, fluid, and relatively quiet motion.

Chapter 5

Time to Get Going!

You're motivated, you're conscientious, you're equipped, and you have learned about proper mechanics. So, are you ready to go running? Or are you wondering where you should begin? If this is your first time running, read on to learn how to run and to review some important tips.

5

Starting Out

Even if you've never run a step in your life, the training schedule on page 57 will enable you to become a runner in a matter of a few short weeks. Where you choose to begin this schedule depends on your current fitness level. If you're just getting into a cardiovascular exercise program, start at the beginning of Week One with brisk walking and proceed through the schedule as indicated. For individuals who currently are quite active (who, at a minimum, can easily walk at a brisk pace and/or jog nonstop for 2 minutes), begin following the schedule at Week Seven.

To minimize your chance of incurring an injury, be patient and stick to the schedule. By all means, avoid the urge to do more than is specified. During the early weeks of the schedule, feel free to break up the cumulative minutes indicated for running into smaller segments if you feel it necessary. There's no problem in modifying the schedule to fit into your busy lifestyle so long as you keep the sequence of runs the same. For example, if Sunday is not a good day for you to run, the time and/or mileage goal indicated on that day can be shifted to another day of the week as long as the sequence for the remainder of runs during the week is also shifted.

The pace of your running should be at an aerobic level (meaning the ability to breathe easily without pushing yourself). In other words, you should be running very relaxed and comfortably. You should be able to talk in complete sentences without gasping for air. If you find yourself huffing and puffing, you are probably running too fast and need to slow down your pace.

In the beginning, the key to success and evaluation of your progress should be based on the cumulative minutes you are able to run without stopping rather than on the pace at which you run. With consistent training over a period of weeks, your running form will become more refined and efficient. This in itself often translates into a faster pace without the need to overload your present musculoskeletal system. Consider running for cumulative time rather than running the same measured route day after day. By doing so, you will stay motivated and thus avoid burnout.

Table 5-1 **Beginner Run/Walk Schedule**

Week #	Sun.	Mon.	Tue.	Wed.	Thur.	Fri.	Sat.	Total
1	W-8	Rest	W-10	Rest	W-11	Rest	W-8	W-37
2	W-12	Rest	W-14	Rest	W-16	Rest	W-10	W-52
3	W-18	Rest	W-20	Rest	W-22	Rest	W-12	W-72
4	W-24	Rest	W-26	Rest	W-28	Rest	W-12	W-90
5	W-30	Rest	W-30	Rest	W-30	Rest	W-30	W-120
6	W-20	Rest	W-20	Rest	W-26	Rest	W-20	W-86 Light Week
7	R-2 W-28	Rest	R-3 W-27	Rest	R-4 W-26	Rest	W-30	R-9 W-81
8	R-5 W-25	Rest	R-6 W-24	Rest	R-8 W-22	Rest	R-6 W-24	R-25 W-95
9	R-10 W-20	Rest	R-11 W-19	Rest	R-12 W-18	Rest	R-8 W-22	R-41 W-79
10	R-14 W-16	Rest	R-16 W-14	Rest	R-18 W-12	Rest	R-10 W-20	R-58 W-62
11	R-20 W-10	Rest	R-22 W-8	Rest	R-24 W-6	Rest	R-12 W-18	R-78 W-42
12	R-26 W-4	Rest	R-28 W-2	Rest	R-30	Rest	R-14 W-16	R-96 W-22
13	R-20 Rest	R-20 W-10	Rest	R-26 W-4	Rest	R-16 W-14	R-82 W-26 Light Week	
14	R-30	Rest	R-25 W-5	Rest	R-30	Rest	R-18 W-12	R-103 W-17
15	R-33	Rest	R-30	Rest	R-30	Rest	R-20 W-10	R-113 W-10
16	R-36	Rest	R-30	Rest	R-30	Rest	R-20 W-10	R-116 W-10
17	R-39	Rest	R-30	Rest	R-30	Rest	R-30	R-129
18	R-20 W-10	Test	R-20 W-010	Rest	R-26 W-4	Rest	R-20 W-10	R-86 W-34 Light Week

W = Walk; R = Run; Numbers = Minutes of exercise

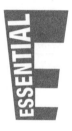

Even if your goal is to run, don't ever be ashamed to walk. In fact, the first sections of the beginner schedule feature a mixture of walking and running. If you are unable to run the specified time and/or mileage goal on the schedule at the present time for whatever reason (aches, pain, fatigue, etc.), then by all means walk the distance.

Learning How to Run

Even if you're a few pounds over your ideal weight or if you haven't exercised in years, if you can walk for 15 or 20 minutes, this schedule can make you a runner. It can also take you to your first 5K in eighteen weeks!

When starting out, have fun, and don't give in to the desire to do too much too soon—or worse, don't quit before you reap the benefits that running can provide. Be patient with yourself and consistent in your workout. In short, enjoy the process, but don't overdo it. Happiness in running comes from the journey, not with the final destination.

Tips Before You Begin

Before you head out the door, review the following tips. Even though running is a simple activity, you need to be mindful of what you're doing at all times in order to maximize its benefits and your enjoyment.

- Be aware of road slants
- Stay hydrated
- Mind the seasons
- Minimize risks
- Let others help

Runners should pay attention to camber, or road slants, regardless of whether they have hip or knee problems. Frequent running on pitched or slanted surfaces increases your chance of incurring injury. If your knees or hips are prone to soreness, you should pay special attention to the camber (the slightly arched shape of the surface of the road or trail) and try to run on the flattest portion. This will reduce the angular stress that can make any injury a more serious problem.

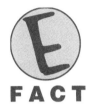

FACT

The shortest distance between two points is a straight line. In training, it is fine to hug the wide lines. But when you are running in a road race or timed event, look for and run the shortest official course, especially on curves and turns. Hugging the outside border of the road can add mileage and time to your performance.

For hot, humid days and for runs of over half an hour, it is very important that you drink fluids every 25 minutes. Above all, don't wait until you're thirsty to start taking in fluids. Before setting out, drink 8 ounces of water and hydrate regularly during your run. For runs lasting an hour or longer, it is important to also consume sports drinks such as Gatorade or Powerade. (See Chapter 3 for more information on carrying systems for fluids that can be secured to one's waist or back, leaving the hands free and not upsetting one's form or comfort.)

You can also plan your route so that you are able to stop at water fountains along the way. As mentioned in Chapter 3, another good idea is to stash bottled water and sports drinks along your course in advance. Lots of runners do this without too much difficulty, and it alleviates the problem of having to carry fluids with you. Doing so also offers the psychological advantage of breaking up the run mentally, since you can set yourself the goal of running from one fluid stop to the next. If you do this, be mindful of the trash this generates. If there aren't trashcans or recycle bins on your route for the empty bottles or drink containers, be sure to go back along the route in a car so you can pick up and properly dispose of your garbage.

Certainly one of the great things about running is that it is a year-round sport. You can run through every season as long as you adequately hydrate and dress appropriately. Dress warmly enough in winter and dress to stay cool enough in summer. Be especially careful on extremely hot or cold days. You should always try to avoid running in extreme heat and extreme cold. If you really must run in such conditions, bring plenty of water with you or place water along the course of your run and consider shortening your workout for that day. (There are more tips about running in hot and cold weather in Chapter 9.)

Cautions

Running, like many other sports, poses its own set of potential problems, including dangers on the trail and risk of injury. One of the most important things you can do is to be aware of your surroundings. Keep your head up and your eyes focused ahead of you rather than down at your feet. If you run in the dark, make yourself visible to others by way of reflective clothing, decals, or tape. Carry a small flashlight so you can see where you are landing.

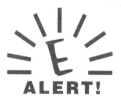

It's important to stay well-hydrated and drink a lot of fluids. But keep in mind that one of the side effects of consuming so many fluids is more frequent trips to the bathroom. Therefore, be sure to use the bathroom before running, especially if you are a morning runner.

Let someone know where you are going, what time you are leaving, and when you expect to return. Why take chances? No matter the distance you plan to run, consider carrying your cell phone so you won't be stranded if you incur injury or need assistance of any type. At the same time, a word to the wise: Don't consider your running time a chance to catch up on phone calls. By cluttering your mind with conversation, you will miss out on the experience of the run. You will also lose focus on your form and your breathing, which is important to maintain if you want to have a beneficial workout. Even though carrying a cell phone is a smart safety feature, resist the temptation to use it unless you have a real emergency.

On a dirt trail, watch out for roots and rocks. Avoid running alone in areas that bears and mountain lions call home. For safety reasons, women should find companions to accompany them when running in unpopulated areas. Dogs and human companions can be fun accompaniments to running, and they provide security against undesired interactions.

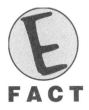

FACT

Different degrees of pain after a workout can include soreness (a light, achy feeling); aches (continuous dull throbbing); and pains (acute and sharp hurting). If soreness or aches don't diminish, take some time off from running. If pain increases, stay off the injury, apply RICE (rest, ice, compress, elevation), and take a pain reliever. If the pain doesn't subside in a few days, see a doctor.

Don't overdo it, especially in the beginning. One of the negative effects of running excessive mileage or running too frequently (that is, not scheduling regular rest days) is the risk of incurring injury. Injuries to the knees, hips, and Achilles tendons, in particular, can often be attributed to overtraining. Listen to your body, and don't make comparisons between your training program and the mileage totals of other runners.

Stay Motivated

Making this change in your life by taking up running is a big deal and something you should feel really good about. Make a copy of whichever training schedule you choose from this book and put it in a prominent place in your home. This way both you and others in your household will be reminded of it. With the schedule clearly displayed, you can chart your progress.

In fact, you can keep yourself motivated by asking your housemates to help you stay on track. That way, when you meet your goals they can share in your success and help celebrate what has become truly a group effort. This might even inspire someone you live with to join you in running.

The advantage of soliciting your housemates' help is that if you miss a day running, others are happy to point it out to you. You wouldn't want to let them (or yourself) down, would you? That's motivation to get back on track and be able to say, "I did it!" the next time they ask.

The disadvantage of involving members if your household is that if you miss a day, and then two, and then three, your spouse and/or kids will still be happy to point it out to you, but if you don't get back on track, you won't want to hear them pestering you about it, and you won't want them to think you may have given up so easily—even if you think you have a great excuse, like you've taken on another committee at school. So think about this before you do it. You may want to keep your progress to yourself and then, one day, invite everyone to the 5K you've entered. Won't they be surprised and delighted!

Working with a Professional

Whether you are a beginner or an experienced competitive runner, there are many reasons to consider a personal training service. These include:

- To begin a running program from square one
- To train to complete short events, from the 5K to half-marathon
- To complete your first marathon safely and successfully
- To improve upon your finish time and conditioning level from a previous race
- To give structure to your training in the face of a busy lifestyle
- To maximize the benefits of training while reducing the chance of injury
- To take your running to the next level

When considering a personal coach, think about what you want from her and understand what you can and can't expect. Typical components of a personal training program include:

- Telephone consultations on a weekly basis
- E-mail support
- Goal-setting assistance
- Individualized training program based on your goals and needs
- Analysis of progress with adjustments based on your results
- Injury prevention guidance
- Nutritional tips
- Answers to your training questions
- Ongoing motivation and support

If you decide to opt for the services of a personal coach, research coaches in your area by talking to other runners, whom you can find through local running clubs.

Beginning Your Running Program

Remember that the safest and most enjoyable approach to running is to build up your ability incrementally. By following the suggestions and schedules in this book, you will find that your ability as a runner increases safely and steadily.

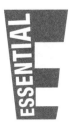

"I've been running since I was in my thirties, and had never broken the barrier from a few minutes to long distance. Until Art Liberman put me on a training program—and it worked. Beginning with 12 minutes, I am now able to run 90-plus minutes nonstop."—Margo Painter, Pensacola, FL

Building a Base

Without question, the most important area one should focus on prior to beginning any running program is safely and slowly building your mileage. In anticipation of entering races longer than 10K (6.2 miles), you should eventually be running four to five days a week with minimum weekly mileage totals of 20–25 miles. You should not introduce advanced running techniques, such as speed work and hill repeats, into your training schedule until you're ready. At that point, longer runs and weekly mileage can be added in small increments.

Going to the Next Level

Assuming you have either completed the walk/run schedule or can run 4 miles prior to picking up this book, you can use the mileage buildup schedule to prepare to run a 10-mile race. If you already have some running experience and wish to enter races longer than 10 miles (such as the half-marathon and marathon) in the near future, put your current training on hold as you complete the last couple of weeks of this schedule.

Prior to your target race, include a taper period of one to two weeks in which you reduce your mileage totals 35–40 percent. By doing so, you will be well rested and ready to perform optimally. Use the walk/run schedule to set the stage for completing your first 5K (rather than for running competitively).

The 10 Percent Rule

Do not increase either your weekly mileage or your long-run mileage by more than 10 percent a week. Doing so greatly increases the chance of incurring an injury, thereby delaying or stopping your training all together. (Refer to Chapter 13 for additional information.) Many running injuries can be attributed to runners not following this simple but extremely important premise.

Table 5-2

Mileage Buildup Schedule

Week #	Sun.	Mon.	Tue.	Wed.	Thur.	Fri.	Sat.	Total
1	4	Rest	3	Rest	4	Test	3	14
2	4	Test	4	Rest	4	Rest	3	15
3	5	Test	4	Rest	4	Rest	3	16
4	3	Rest	3	Rest	3	Rest	3	12 Light Week
5	5	Rest	4	Rest	4	Rest	4	17
6	6	Rest	4	Rest	4	Rest	4	18
7	6	Rest	4	Rest	5	Rest	4	19
8	3	Rest	4	Rest	3	Rest	3	13 Light Week
9	7	Rest	4	Rest	5	Rest	4	20
10	7	Rest	5	Rest	5	Rest	4	21
11	8	Rest	5	Rest	5	Rest	4	22
12	4	Rest	3	Rest	4	Rest	4	15 Light Week
13	8	Rest	5	Rest	6	Rest	4	23
14	9	Rest	5	Rest	6	Rest	4	24
15	9	Rest	6	Rest	6	Rest	4	25
16	5	Rest	4	Rest	4	Rest	4	17 Light Week
17	10	Rest	6	Rest	6	Rest	4	26
18	10	Rest	6	Rest	7	Rest	4	27
19	6	Rest	4	Rest	5	Rest	4	19 Light Week

Numbers refer to miles of running

Table 5-3

Advanced Mileage Buildup Schedule

Week #	Sun.	Mon.	Tue.	Wed.	Thur.	Fri.	Sat.	Total
1	4	Rest	3	Rest	4	Rest	3	14
2	4	Rest	4	Rest	4	Rest	3	15
3	5	Rest	4	Rest	4	Rest	3	16
4	3	Rest	3	Rest	3	Rest	3	12 Light Week
5	5	Rest	3	3	3	Rest	3	17
6	6	Rest	3	3	3	Rest	3	18
7	6	Rest	3	4	3	Rest	4	20
8	3	Rest	4	Rest	3	Rest	3	13 Light Week
9	7	Rest	3	5	4	Rest	3	22
10	7	Rest	4	5	4	Rest	4	24
11	8	Rest	4	6	4	Rest	4	26
12	4	Rest	3	Rest	4	Rest	4	15 Light Week
13	8	Rest	5	6	5	Rest	4	28
14	9	Rest	5	5	6	Rest	4	29
15	9	Rest	5	7	6	Rest	5	32
16	5	Rest	4	Rest	4	Rest	4	17 Light Week
17	10	Rest	6	8	6	Rest	4	34
18	10	Rest	6	8	7	Rest	4	35
19	6	Rest	4	Rest	5	Rest	4	19 Light Week

Numbers refer to miles of running

Beginning Runner's Mistakes

Watch out for common mistakes that beginning runners often make. These include:

- **Focusing on speed.** Try to focus on increasing your duration rather than your speed as a means of evaluating your progress.
- **Doing too much too soon.** Increasing mileage as a result of over-enthusiasm often leads to the most common beginner running injury—shin splints (see Chapter 15).
- **Not listening to your body.** If excessively sore or fatigued, either walk or take an extra day off.
- **Using old running shoes or shoes not designed specifically for running.** Run in shoes that are biomechanically appropriate to your body's running needs.
- **Training with the wrong people.** Run with others who share your level of ability, not with those who run either much faster or slower than you.
- **Trying to emulate other people's running styles.** Use the proper form when you run to avoid discomfort or injury.
- **Giving up too soon.** If you find yourself getting discouraged soon after you start a running program, be careful not to talk yourself out of it. Go back to Chapters 1 and 2 and reevaluate the reasons you wanted to start running. Ask yourself what happened between having those feelings and becoming discouraged. Are your expectations unrealistic? Is there something about the process that doesn't feel right? Do you recognize any mistakes listed here as contributing to your feeling discouraged?

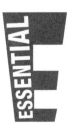

"Physically, I feel great and have gotten my 'gut' back into running. I recently set a personal record, running a half-marathon here in 1:35:45. Overall, I feel very strong and confident. I couldn't have made it to this point without your advice and guidance, and again, for that, I thank you."—Ann Marie C., Chicago, IL

A More Advanced Schedule

When you complete your choice of buildup schedule, you will have developed a base from which you can now train for race distances longer than 10 miles. The advanced mileage buildup schedule features five days of training (on most weeks) and more weekly mileage than the previous mileage buildup schedule.

So how do you decide which schedule to choose? Some readers of this book are already at or above the level of the basic buildup schedule and will want other mileage buildup options. These runners have the time and desire to train five days a week. If this describes you, make sure you are up to it and can comfortably train at this level. Don't push yourself too hard by selecting a schedule that does not yet match your present level of conditioning.

At the conclusion of Week Nineteen of either schedule, assuming that you've made it through the mileage buildup stage without injury, you are now ready to proceed to new training goals. These might include incorporating more advanced training techniques (such as speed work) and/or training for longer races such as the half-marathon and marathon.

Chapter 6

Ready for Racing: The 5K

The 5K offers all levels of runners an array of challenges. Experienced runners may wish to improve their time from a previous race, whereas beginning runners might simply hope to finish the event. Regardless of your motivation, running the 5K is a goal that you can accomplish after just a few short weeks of training. By the time you complete the first training schedule, you'll be able to at least finish a 5K without months of intense preparation, even if you have to walk for part or all of it.

5K Basics

Today the 5K (5 kilometers) is a distance that's familiar to runners the world over. It is accepted internationally as the introductory distance for novice runners as well as the proving ground for more competitive runners (and every level in between). Its distance—3.1 miles—doesn't seem that long and isn't too difficult to train for. But like most things that appear simple at first, the 5K is a race distance that challenges even elite runners to return for more.

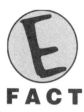

FACT

The larger 5K races across the United States typically include at least one vendor of running gear. These are good venues to find sales on the basics: shorts, socks, and even shoes. You can reward yourself for competing in the event by supplementing your running wardrobe before you go home.

You will find that 5K events are a lot of fun. The races are usually well-organized and are often supported by corporate sponsors, area businesses, a running club, or perhaps a local booster organization. These races are like little running fairs. Participants sometimes receive T-shirts, samples of running foods and other running products, as well as a wealth of information about other races in the vicinity of the running locale.

Also attendant at many 5Ks are small, local running specialty stores that feature wares such as new running shoes, running apparel, and other running-related accessories. It is not uncommon for people to have some fun indulging in a little shopping either before or after the race.

Of course, you'll also see a lot of other runners at 5K events. They come alone, in pairs, or in groups, all from diverse backgrounds. Buddies, girlfriends, boyfriends, couples, and families all attend, and they all love running as well as socializing with fellow runners.

Race Strategy and Goal Setting

Goal setting is indeed important. Not only does it keep your training in focus, but it makes competing in races both fun and challenging. In the weeks prior to the race, think about three goals you'd be interested in accomplishing: an easily obtainable goal, a realistic yet moderately challenging goal, and an ultimate goal. Be realistic. For example, if you don't posses the genetic gift to run a sub-16-minute 5K, don't set that as your ultimate goal.

Some 5K goals include completing the entire event running, improving your time by 30 seconds to 1 full minute, or coming in under a specific time. By making sure these goals are realistic, you will avoid being disappointed and instead be satisfied or even thrilled with your performance. Above all, it's important to keep the event in perspective. Sure, races are competitive. Sure, you want to do your best. But remember that one of the great things about running is that you're ultimately competing with yourself. So keep a healthy perspective, give yourself an achievable goal, and keep the fun in the 5K.

The Week Before Your 5K

There is no workout you can do in the last week prior to your 5K that will enhance your performance. Therefore, make the final week prior to the big race an easy one with light workouts (continue to follow either of the mileage buildup charts in Chapter 5). Make one of the two days prior to the event a complete leg rest day.

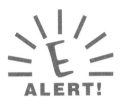

ALERT!

Don't try anything radically new or different in the weeks before your 5K. Don't try a new diet; don't try new shoes. Taper your mileage at an easy pace, get adequate rest, and prepare yourself mentally for the big day.

Don't break with your training schedule or try anything radically different the week before your race either. For example, one of the most frequent mistakes that comes back to haunt the unsuspecting runner, whether it be in a short event or in a marathon, is to run in new shoes purchased the day before the race. It takes at least a few training runs for new shoes to get broken in. Wearing new shoes even a few days before the race can cause a variety of problems, such as blister and foot discomfort, which affects your performance in the race.

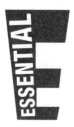

Lay out everything you need (apparel, shoes, etc.) the evening before the race to save yourself time, stress, and aggravation in the morning. You don't want to be halfway there and realize you've forgotten something, especially if you have to help others get ready to go with you. It's important to have everything you need arranged ahead of time.

What to Eat and Drink

Nutrition principles dictate that you should always stay well-hydrated, whether you are exercising or not. In particular, drink ample fluids in the days prior to competition, regardless of how long the race may be, what the weather is like the day of the race, whether the course is particularly hilly, or other conditions of the race.

For workouts and races that last an hour or less, you need only drink water every 25–30 minutes to stay well-hydrated. Although sports drinks do play an important role during runs lasting an hour and longer, they won't necessarily give you a performance edge for shorter workouts and events such as the 5K. Consuming sports drinks can be especially helpful when training in hot and humid conditions, however, as they refuel your body's electrolyte stores.

Eating Before Race Day

Carbohydrate loading and eating in general is a major consideration in running, whether to fuel your body for training runs or a road race. However, you really don't need to load up too much on carbohydrates the day or two before a 5K, not in the same way you do for a marathon.

Don't stuff yourself, thinking you're just going to burn off the calories the next day. And don't eat new foods you haven't eaten during your training. Many a runner has rued the time he decided to have exotic or unfamiliar food the day before a race. Eat something you know will agree with you. Otherwise, regardless of your pace, the consequence of poor nutritional choice can be discomforting and perhaps even embarrassing.

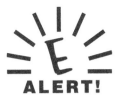

ALERT!

If you're like most runners, you live for your next meal. Well, plan your eating extravagance for the night after the 5K. Leading up to the event, be mindful of any unnecessary fat, sugar, or other nutritional bombs that might put you in the Port-a-John instead of on the starting line the day of the race.

In summary, your evening meal the day before the race should consist of well-balanced and simple foods that you know will cause no digestive troubles. A mix of 65 percent carbohydrates, 20 percent protein, and 15 percent fat is optimal. Avoid foods that are high in salt, fat, or fried. You also want to limit your intake of foods with high roughage content, such as salads, vegetables, and cereals.

Drinking Before Race Day

As stressed throughout this book, stay well-hydrated. If you enjoy beverages that contain caffeine such as coffee or tea, be aware that drinking these in late afternoon or evening may make it difficult for you to fall asleep easily, especially if you've got pre-race jitters. Additionally, caffeinated as well as alcoholic beverages are diuretics that can contribute to dehydration.

At the other extreme, if you're taking in excessive fluids through water or sports drinks, you may experience hyponatremia, or water intoxication, a condition in which excess fluids create an imbalance between the body's water and sodium levels. This can lead to nausea, fatigue, vomiting, or worse. (Learn more about hyponatremia in Chapter 16.)

Eating on Race Day

Equally important is your decision regarding what to eat on race day. If the race is set for early in the morning (as most 5Ks are), you may wish to bypass breakfast and just stick with water. If you choose to eat a light snack (this could be a banana, slice of toast, bagel, or energy bar), be sure to consume it at least 1 hour before the start of the race.

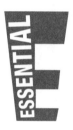

Try to go to bed early the night prior to the race so that you will be well rested for the event. You don't want to be rushed or, worse, oversleep and miss the race. Wake up early enough to eat, make a visit to the bathroom, and take care of anything you need to do so as not to feel rushed.

Events held during the late morning, midafternoon, or evening are more difficult to plan for nutritionally. While you certainly don't want to go hungry in the hours prior to a race or a fast-paced workout, you don't want to eat foods that cause stomach cramps or digestive problems.

Light, healthy snacks are your best approach for late morning and early afternoon races. If the race will be held in the evening, eat a healthy and satisfying breakfast along with a sensible but light lunch (avoid high-fat and fried foods). A piece of fruit or a handful of pretzels are good snack choices later in the afternoon. In short, the best way to determine which foods and fluids work best for you, whether during training runs or races, is by experimenting with these in practice.

Physical Preparation

Listen to your body. As mentioned previously, there are no workouts the week prior to any distance race that can enhance your preparedness. A general rule of thumb is that less is best. The physiological effects of training don't kick in for a week to ten days, so the workout you do today will not immediately enhance your level of performance.

Remember also not to try anything new the week prior to and during your 5K. There are so many heartbreaking stories of runners who tried something new in the week prior to a race, only to injure themselves and not be able to participate in the event at all. Don't let that happen to you.

The following are some 5K pre-race reminders:

- Preregister for the event to save time and money.
- Remember that the race will begin on time and regardless of almost any weather conditions (except perhaps lightning storms).
- Arrive at the race site early.
- Pin your race number on the front of your shirt or singlet.
- For races that are computer timed, be sure that your computer chip is attached securely to your running shoe (for example, on an eyelet or on laces located midway down the tongue).

Psychological Issues and Concerns

Remember that it is normal to be tense or nervous prior to a road race of any distance. Even the most seasoned runners experience these feelings. To help yourself stay calm and focused, avoid spending too much time with participants who are excessively stressed out or negative. These individuals may adversely affect your state of mind—something you certainly don't need. If you find being in the company of others prior to an event comforting, gravitate toward those who appear focused and relaxed. Some runners find it calming to spend a few moments alone. Through racing you'll figure out what works best for you.

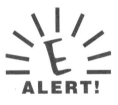

Don't overpack when going to a race. Between the freebies you're given at the race and the goods you'll want to buy, you may have a lot to carry. If you're walking to the race, take a small bag that can be checked at the start. If you drive to the race, you can put your items in your car.

Prior to the start of the event, you'll notice a variety of pre-race activity. You'll see some runners stretching, some doing pre-race warm-up running, some taking in extra fluids. Don't second-guess yourself and think you should be doing any of these for a competitive advantage. If you try doing something different from your tried-and-true warm-up routine because you see others doing it, it may backfire on you during the race. Relax, do what you've rehearsed during your training, and feel good about it.

During the Race

As you are running the 5K, it's easy to get caught up in the excitement of it all. Just be sure that you keep the following essential guidelines in mind to ensure you have the best experience possible.

The Start

When runners line up in anticipation at the start of a 5K (or any race), they are supposed to position themselves in the pack based on their anticipated pace. For example, faster runners—especially those trying to place if not win—line up in front to be sure they get off to as fast a start as possible. Runners with no competitive aspirations or those who are participating strictly for fun should take their place toward the back.

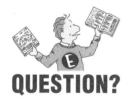

QUESTION?

What if you get injured during the race?
If you feel a significant increase in pain as you continue to run, seriously consider dropping out of the race. No race is worth the risk of hurting yourself by continuing to run and causing a minor injury to turn into a major setback.

Although runners are generally honest people, this protocol does not always hold when they are asked to line up for the start of a race according to their anticipated pace. Unfortunately, too many slower runners line up in front of the faster runners. In addition to this not being fair, in a large race the slower runners can actually create problems (as people tend to be pushed down or slip and fall).

If you're not sure where to line up and are worried about whether you'll get stuck behind the slow runners or quickly left behind by the fast ones, play it safe and head for the middle of the pack. There will be runners who quickly pass you and others that you will pass, but if you're new to running races, this is the best position from which to find your rhythm and enjoy the run. Take a deep breath and know that you are going to have fun, stay relaxed, and achieve your goals.

Pacing and Staying Relaxed

Running at the appropriate pace for your ability level is crucial for all distances, from sprints to the marathon, to enhance your chance of performing optimally and therefore running your fastest possible race. It is so easy to start the race running much faster than you should—and you may not even realize it! Your pace during the first mile may feel effortless due to the adrenaline rush and excitement of the event. But speed can cause you to burn out by the second or third mile.

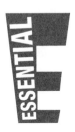

Something you'll probably see all the runners around you doing is readying their watches prior to the start of the race. You should do the same. Be prepared so that when you hear, "Runners take your mark, set, go!" your watch is already at zero and all you have to do is push the start button to be on pace.

Be sure to check your watch at the mile markers of the race (called mile splits) to see how off the official time you may be. The information you get from your watch as well as the split times called by the people manning the mile markers can both help you stay on pace.

For races in which many runners compete, the organization holding the event may use computer chips to time the runners. The chips activate at the starting line and stop at the finish. If you're toward the back of a pack in such a race, don't start your watch when the officials shout "Go!" since it might take you a while to reach the actual starting line and your time will be thrown off. Instead, start your watch at the starting line and look at it at each mile marker. The split times shouted out by the people manning the markers may not be what you're running either, because their time started when the announcer said "Go!" Working your watch this way during a big race is the only way you'll know with any sense of accuracy your true pace mile by mile, as well as your actual finish time immediately after the race.

Running each mile at the same pace is a proven approach to turning in your best race time. If you feel like you're really overextending yourself, you probably are. Taper back a bit and see whether you feel like catching some folks at the end. You'll enjoy finishing strong.

Another way to avoid draining your energy too quickly is to remember to stay loose and relaxed. Be sure to shake out your arms and shoulders occasionally throughout the race to avoid upper body muscle tightness. This will contribute to a more comfortable run.

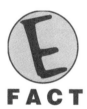

FACT

Chances are you'll run faster in a race than you do during your training runs, even if your goal is not to go faster. The rush of the crowd and the fact that it's a race contribute to the excitement, which usually translates into a faster pace.

Water Stops and Supplements

Most races have water stops, at which eager volunteers hold out cups of water for you to take as you pass. Mastering the art of drinking while you're running takes some practice. But the only way to do it is to, well, do it. So give it a try. If you're not too successful and get most of the water on your face or shirt, oh well. What you don't want to do is inhale the water and end up choking. So if it's easier and more comfortable for you, just slow down to a walk for a few steps while you drink.

If it's a really hot day, you can also pour water over your head, on your neck, chest, and hands. As for supplements like energy gels or a sports beverage, you don't really need them in a 5K.

After the Race

Congratulations, you did it! Savor the excitement of finishing, no matter when you came in. Then, after crossing the line, get something to drink. Within a few minutes of finishing, do a 5–10 minute cool-down jog to begin the recovery process. Stretch thoroughly immediately after the race. Doing so will keep muscle soreness to a minimum over the next day or two. And, of course, chat about the race with your fellow runners.

When you get home, look at the flyers you collected at the race to consider when and where to run your next 5K (or maybe an even longer race). If you're like most runners, you'll be hooked on the exhilarating feeling of having successfully competed in the race.

Chapter 7

Stretching and Weight Training

Stretching is an extremely important part of running. Stretching keeps your muscles from cramping and reduces the possibility of injury. It helps to lengthen your muscles and improve your flexibility. In the end, it will improve and lengthen stride and increase your overall speed and stamina. Weight training, like stretching, can enhance your running by both improving your performance and reducing your chances of incurring injury. By increasing muscle mass you can improve abdominal, back, arm, and leg strength. This chapter examines how to incorporate both these valuable practices into your running routine.

Helping Your Muscles Help You

The human body is an amazing machine, and muscles are a large part of what drives it. There are about 650 muscles in the body, and they provide all kinds of support and propulsion. The skeletal muscles, in conjunction with tendons and ligaments, support the body's frame and give it shape; smooth muscles line body organs; and cardiac muscles pump the heart. Muscles are working all the time to adjust your posture, move your body parts, help keep you upright, operate certain bodily functions, and generate heat in your body.

Skeletal muscles work in pairs so that when you move, while one contracts, another relaxes. This way, all the parts that need to bend can also return to their normal position. Muscles need the nutrients and oxygen from blood to keep them functioning. Nutrition and exercise affect these very important parts of your body; the better muscles are cared for, the better they perform.

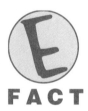

FACT

Skeletal muscles are made up of very elastic fibers connected by tissue. Each fiber develops from the fusion of many cells specific to the function of the muscle. Blood vessels and nerves run through the connective tissue. Skeletal muscle fibers line up in bands and are called *striated* muscles.

Done properly, exercise strengthens muscles, helping them to do their job better. If you exacerbate a muscle group because you overwork it (even without intending to), you can strain and even tear your muscles, which can force you to stop exercising until the muscles heal. To avoid this, you want to treat your muscles with respect. Warm them up, don't push them too hard, and help strengthen them properly by stretching carefully and thoroughly.

Stretch After You Run

A major misconception about running is that you must stretch beforehand. In fact, the opposite is the case: You should stretch after a workout. If you really feel you should stretch because you want to loosen up or warm up your muscles before the serious work, jog or walk for 5–10 minutes and then stretch. The best thing to do is to start your run very slowly, then ease into a training pace 5–10 minutes later. The idea is not to stretch a cold muscle. If you're planning to do a speed workout or race, jog for about a mile, stretch, do striders (see later in this chapter), and then do the speed workout or race.

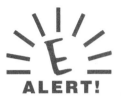

Before stretching, you need to warm up your muscles. Don't stretch past the point of slight discomfort. If your muscles are still cold, don't try to stretch them like a rubber band, especially if you haven't run in a while.

It's very important to remember to stretch after a run. A workout isn't over until, as part of your cool-down period, you stretch thoroughly immediately following the run. You need to make sure you establish the good work habits of successful runners, for whom the stretching period after the run is as important as the run itself.

View stretching as a part of your overall workout. It should be just as natural and routine as jogging to warm up before an event. This is because your legs are most receptive to the benefits of stretching immediately after you run. Stretching 30–40 minutes later when your muscles have cooled down actually increases your chances of causing injury. Your muscles are fatigued and tight after a run, especially after a long or fast-paced one, and stretching can help to alleviate soreness later.

In short, stretch gently and slowly while your muscles are still warm. One final rule: No bouncing when you stretch. That is called ballistic stretching, and it can cause injuries!

Stretching Fundamentals

Whenever you stretch, remember the objectives of stretching, which are to improve flexibility, strengthen and lengthen your muscles so they can perform optimally, prevent injuries, and enhance circulation. When you integrate stretching into your overall workout routine, you'll be amazed by how much better you'll feel all over.

How to Stretch Properly

Have you ever seen someone go about stretching haphazardly? He throws his foot onto a fence post or railing, awkwardly bends toward it, bounces a few times, tries to grab his foot a couple of times, then heaves his foot back down and starts with the other one. Common sense says there's something wrong with this all-too-common sight, and indeed there is.

To be effective, stretching needs to be slow, gentle, and focused. Concentrate on the muscles or muscle groups you're working on and breathe naturally and regularly (no holding your breath). Inhale as you set up the stretch, then exhale as you lean into the stretch, moving slowly and lightly to extend the muscle to its greatest point of extension. Stop when you feel mild tension and hold the stretch for 30–60 seconds. At the end of that time, inhale out of the stretch as gently as you went into it.

Patience Is a Virtue

Even if you currently have poor flexibility, a regular stretching program will greatly improve your range of motion. The key is to be both patient and consistent. Your stretching should not cause pain, although it may feel a bit awkward or even uncomfortable at first when extending a muscle to the far end of its present range of motion.

You can also supplement your stretching with exercises that strengthen your muscles to further support your joints and skeleton. For example, strengthening your abdominals by doing crunches and sit-ups correctly and building up your arms and shoulders using free weights or machines such as Nautilus or Cybex are ways you can benefit your overall health and improve your running. (Learn more in the weight-training section later in this chapter.)

Static stretch basics include:

- Stretch the muscle to the point of its greatest range of motion, but don't overextend.
- Never bounce when stretching; rather, hold the stretch for 30–60 seconds.
- Stretch all the major leg muscle groups.
- Stretch uniformly (after stretching one leg, stretch the other).
- Don't overstretch an injured area, for this may cause additional damage.

The Best Stretches for Runners

The stretches described here benefit the major muscles in your legs—those that support your shins, thighs, ankles, knees, hips, and buttocks.

Stretching the Hamstring

Your hamstrings are located in the backs of your thighs. When they're too tight, you may experience lower back pain. To stretch them out, stand with your feet shoulder-width apart and pointing straight ahead. Start to bend over at the waist, moving your hands together toward your feet. Keep your knees slightly bent as you do this and only go as far down as it takes to feel a minimal tightness.

As you bend down, relax your neck and shoulders and slowly exhale. When you reach the slightly tight point, relax into it and hold for approximately 30 seconds. When the time is up, start straightening back up as you inhale. Move slowly, and allow your head to roll up gently as well. When you're back in the standing position, exhale. Inhale as you begin to bend forward again.

Repeat this stretch 3–5 times. If you do this after every run, you'll notice improvements in your flexibility within a week. Soon you'll be able to reach your knees, then your ankles, and—yes—your toes!

Quadriceps, Knees, and Iliotibial Band

Until you develop the leg strength, you should do this stretch while holding onto or leaning against something for support. To stretch your right quads and iliotibial (IT) band, support yourself with your right hand. Bend your right knee while grabbing your foot with your left hand. With your toes slightly pointed, gently bring your foot toward your buttocks as you exhale. Hold the stretch for about 30 seconds. Switch legs. Repeat until you've stretched both legs 3–4 times. You can also work on improving your balance with this stretch by steadying yourself on the leg you're standing on and removing your hand from the wall or railing.

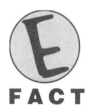

FACT

The *quadriceps* (quads) and *iliotibial band* (IT band) support the knees during exercise. Quads are the muscles in the front of your thigh; the IT band runs from your hip to your knee along the outside of your leg. The stronger these muscles are, the better they can support your knees.

The Lower Body All-Over Stretch

Stand with your feet shoulder-width apart and your toes pointing out slightly. Keeping your feet flat, start to lower yourself into a squat. Exhale. Your knees should be outside of your shoulders but over your big toes. Support yourself with your arms in front of you and between your legs, hands touching the floor (if possible). You may want to do this with your back against a wall for additional support.

When you're squatting, hold the stretch for about 30 seconds. Come up slowly, inhaling as you straighten. Repeat 2–3 times when you're first learning this stretch. As you get better, hold it for a bit longer, and see if you can repeat it 4–5 times.

Stretching the Hips

The hip flexor can help keep you flexible through the hips. Sitting with your legs crossed in front of you, use both arms to take the foot and knee of one leg and stretch them toward you, cradling your leg. Hold for about 30 seconds, and switch legs. Repeat a few times with each leg.

A Simple, Effective Stretching Routine

Stretching is something runners tend to skip, either because they never get into the routine of doing it or they feel they are doing it incorrectly. To avoid being one of these runners, use this simple routine of 4 stretches that can be done in about 10 minutes.

First, stretch out your hamstrings. Lying on your back with your legs extended, bend one leg and bring your knee up toward your chest. Use both hands to hold your leg into your chest. Grasp your leg as far down as you can, making it a goal to be able to grab your foot as you hold the stretch. Hold for approximately 30 seconds, switch legs, and work toward 4–5 repetitions, alternating legs.

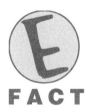

FACT

The squat stretch is a great stretch for your lower back, ankles, Achilles tendons, shins, and groin. If you spend a lot of time sitting or standing, you'll come to love this stretch. However, if you're a beginner, it can be particularly tough—go easy!

Next you will stretch your hips. Shift from lying down to sitting, and do the hip flexor stretch described previously.

After the hip flex, you will stretch your quadriceps. Move from a sitting to a standing position. Lean against a wall or hold a firm rail for support. Then follow the directions for stretching quadriceps described previously in this chapter.

Finally, you will stretch the Achilles tendon, calf, and IT band. Standing with your feet shoulder-width apart, lean forward with your hands out against a wall, tree, or rail so that your body is at a forty-five degree angle. Keep both feet flat on the ground. Lean into the stretch, feeling it in the back of your leg and through your ankle.

Weight Training to Enhance Running

Whether you are young or old, heavy or lean, a long-distance runner or a sprinter, you will benefit from weight training, also known as strength training. The increase in lean muscle mass that results from strength training is key to overall strength and to your body's ability to burn calories. This is because muscle cells require more energy (and also burn more calories) than fat cells.

After the age of thirty, people's muscle mass gradually begins to diminish. As this occurs, people notice that they can no longer eat all they used to without gaining body fat. You may weigh less at age forty-five than you did at thirty-five, but body-composition testing might indicate that you are carrying more body fat than at a younger age. Incorporating strength training three times or so per week in one's personal schedule can slow this process considerably.

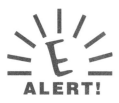

ALERT!

If you have any medical problems, such as heart disease, diabetes, or high blood pressure, or if you are over forty, see your doctor before beginning strength training. If you have carpal tunnel syndrome or any other upper extremity physical problem, you should also consult your physician prior to beginning a strength training program.

Overall fitness requires more than just cardiovascular fitness. A balance of endurance, strength, and flexibility must be achieved. The most often recognized components of fitness include:

- Muscular fitness, strength, and endurance
- Flexibility
- Cardiovascular endurance
- Balanced nutrition
- Body composition

The last item, body composition, acts as a guide to how your body is doing overall, as it takes into account the percentages of fat, bone, and muscle in the body giving the greatest overall assessment. It is not a pure component of fitness. Although running is one of the best cardiovascular activities, other than strengthening a few specific muscles and rapidly burning a lot of calories, it does not fulfill many of the other criteria of overall fitness. That is why weight training is essential to your overall health.

Upper Body Benefits of Weight Training

A strong upper body enables a runner to maintain form late in a marathon or a long run. Additionally, upper body strength reduces fatigue and stiffness in the arms, shoulders, and neck areas. Strong arms and shoulders are helpful in propelling a runner uphill. Finally, legs move only as fast as the arm swings. Thus, a runner with a strong upper body runs faster and more efficiently.

Leg Benefits of Weight Training

Running creates a muscular imbalance in the legs. Through running, one's hamstrings and calf muscles develop at a faster rate than the quadriceps and shins. Weight training helps address this imbalance. Additionally, strong quadriceps and hips help protect these areas from a variety of injuries. Strong legs also offer protection from the possibility of injury when running fast downhill.

Other Benefits of Weight Training

Weight training also helps protect bones. This is an important benefit, particularly for women, because decreased estrogen production causes bone demineralization, which in turn increases the risk of osteoporosis and stress fractures. The gentle pulling action of muscles on bone that happens during weight training facilitates bone regeneration.

Weight training may also help prevent life-threatening illnesses. Some studies show that strength training seems to reduce the risk factors for adult-onset diabetes as well as heart disease.

Upper Body Versus Lower Body

Although many athletes train the entire body with equal intensity and use heavy weights for their legs, heavy strength training for the legs is not necessarily vital or helpful for the long-distance runner. Elite athletes and advanced competitive runners engage in strength training that emphasizes the upper body during their training. Following their example, go easy on the legs, using strength training cautiously (using low weights with a high number of repetitions) while emphasizing upper body work.

As some runners age, they find that more lower extremity exercises are helpful. Some of them have then generalized that if these are good for the aging athlete, they are good for the younger one, too. That is not necessarily so. Younger athletes aren't losing muscle by 5 to 20 percent; they are still in their prime. Young runners are probably better off performing only a light

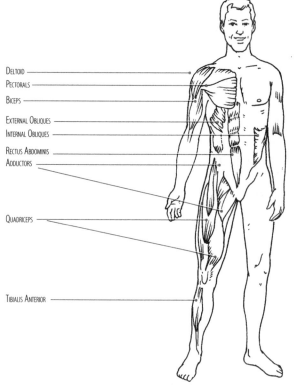

DELTOID
PECTORALS
BICEPS
EXTERNAL OBLIQUES
INTERNAL OBLIQUES
RECTUS ABDOMINIS
ADDUCTORS
QUADRICEPS
TIBIALIS ANTERIOR

Our muscles: front view

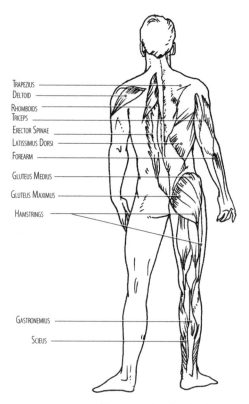

TRAPEZIUS
DELTOID
RHOMBOIDS
TRICEPS
ERECTOR SPINAE
LATISSIMUS DORSI
FOREARM
GLUTEUS MEDIUS
GLUTEUS MAXIMUS
HAMSTRINGS
GASTRONEMIUS
SCLEUS

Our muscles: back view

lower extremity workout in combination with different running techniques to enhance their running speed, form, and strength. Such techniques, discussed in greater depth in Chapter 11, include fartlek workouts, striders, hill repeats, tempo runs, and repeat intervals.

Of course, there is value to gentle leg extensions, leg presses, leg curls, straight leg lifts, and (sometimes) gentle calf raises, as well as crunches. Just don't go overboard on the muscles that runners exercise the most.

Since you're going to be working muscles you might not have known you even had, the following is a brief anatomy lesson to help you both identify and appreciate your muscles. Knowing where the muscles are located and what they do enables you to understand what you're working out and why.

Shoulders, Back, and Chest

A variety of muscles work together in your shoulders, back, and chest. The muscles that traverse your chest below your breasts are called *pectorals* but are commonly referred to as pecs. Stretching along the tops of your arms near your shoulders are your *deltoids*. Nearby are your *rotator cuffs*, a group of four muscles under your shoulder that are used for carrying, catching, and throwing. The *trapezius* is a diamond-shaped muscle that runs across the shoulders, toward the neck, and into the lower back.

In your back, you'll find the *erector spinae,* the muscles that run the length of the spine and that flex to straighten, bend, sit, stand, and lie down. Also running down your back is the *latissimus dorsi,* a large muscle that goes from below your shoulder to your lower back. In the center of your back are triangular-shaped muscles known as *rhomboids,* which keep the shoulder blades together and assist in proper posture.

Arms and Abs

The muscles of your arms and midsection are also important. In your arms, the *biceps* are the muscles on the front of your arm, the ones you flex when someone asks to see how strong you are. The companion muscles to the biceps are the *triceps.* These are located on the back of your upper arm.

On the midsection, you will find your *obliques* and *rectus abdominis.* There are internal and external obliques that line both sides of your midsection and support the rectus abdominis. Meanwhile, rectus abdominis muscles extend from below the chest to just below the navel. They are more commonly referred to as abs.

Hips, Butt, and Legs

Essential to runners, the major lower body muscles are the *gluteus maximus, gluteus medius,* and *gluteus minimus,* all of which are commonly called gluts. Other lower body muscles include the *hamstrings* (a group of three muscles at the back of the thigh) and the *quadriceps* (a group of four muscles on the front of the thigh). You should also be aware of the *tibialis anterior,* a group of muscles that extends along your *tibia* (the bone that goes from your knee to your ankle, along the shin).

Practical Weight Training

Since this is a running book, the weight training exercises included here are ones that you can do at home and that give you all the benefits described above. Although these exercises don't necessitate your going to the gym, if you want to take this training to the next level, go for it! Work with someone knowledgeable at the gym so you are using the appropriate amount of weight to work the muscles you want to target. And remember what was said about overworking your legs—it's not a good idea.

Types of Weights to Use

If you're starting as a complete beginner, the best weights to use are dumbbells, which you can buy at a sporting goods store. Dumbbells are convenient, portable, and not overwhelming. You can use them while watching television or talking on the phone. They come in various weights, and you'll need a few so you can use different ones to work different muscles. If the only upper body work you've done is lifting utensils to eat and drink, you probably want to start out with 3-pound weights. You'll graduate to 5 pounds in a few weeks and may be ready to work with 10-pound weights in a few months.

You may also want to purchase weights for lower body work. A handy type of weight to use for leg strengthening is the kind that goes around your ankle and is adjusted with a Velcro strap. Again, be sure not to overdo it with leg exercises!

Using Weights

There are two ways to hold your dumbbells: overhand and underhand. For the overhand grip, grab the dumbbell with your palm facing down and knuckles facing up. For the underhand grip, your palm should be facing up and your knuckles down.

There are two ways to stand as well. One is with your feet shoulder-width apart, head and shoulders level, back erect, and knees slightly bent. This is the standard stand. The other position is bent over, feet shoulder-width apart, with one leg slightly extended. The idea is to work with a flat back and with your nonworking arm resting on the same-side thigh.

When first beginning a strength training program, you should only perform one set of each exercise for the first couple of weeks, doing 12 to 15 repetitions (reps) of an exercise. Don't feel overwhelmed and think you must increase the number of sets to reap strength training benefits. After this, you may increase to 2 or 3 sets after 1 warm-up set. If you feel as if you could go well beyond 15–20 reps, increase the weight on your next set or at your next session.

Upper Body Exercises

Your upper body workout should target the upper body muscles described above. Remember, for maximum results, use the appropriate weight (the weight at which you can do no more than 12–15 reps).

Biceps Curl and Triceps Kickback

From the standing position, arms at your side, hold the dumbbell with an underhand grip. With your elbow securely against your side, raise (curl) the dumbbell up and toward your chest as far as it will go, then control the

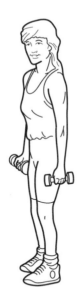
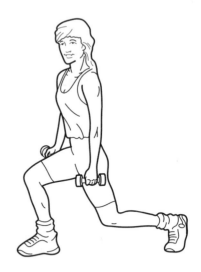

Starting position for the biceps curl

Finishing position for the biceps curl

weight as you bring your hand back down. This is one repetition. Alternate arms after each set.

For the triceps kickback, use an overhand grip and, in the bent-over position, extend the working arm straight behind you (kick it back) without hyperextending your arm. Control the weight as you bend back toward your chest. This is one repetition.

Front Raise and Shoulder Press

The front raise works your deltoids. In the standing position with the dumbbell in an overhand grip, let both arms rest in front of your body so that your palms are resting on your thighs. Then lift one arm straight up to shoulder height so that it's parallel to the floor. Control the weight on the way back to the starting position for one repetition.

For the shoulder press, stand with the dumbbells in an overhand grip, bend your arms so that the dumbbells are by your ears, palms facing away

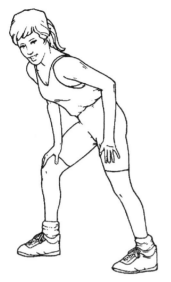

Bent-over position for the triceps kickback

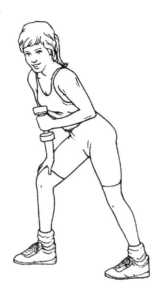

Starting position for the triceps kickback

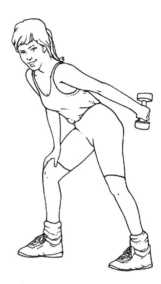

Finish position for the triceps kickback

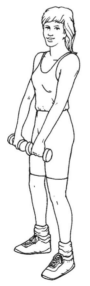

Start position for the front raise

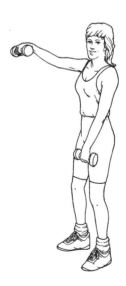

Finish position for the front raise

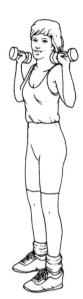

Start position for the shoulder
press

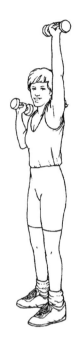

Finish position for the shoulder
press

from your body. Extend your arm up and slightly in front of your head, then lower to the starting position for one rep.

Bent-Over Row

From the bent-over position, hold the dumbbell in an overhand grip and extend your arm toward the floor in a diagonal line from your shoulder. As if you are rowing a boat, bend your elbow and lift the dumbbell so that you use your back muscles as well as your arm muscles. Pretend you're starting a lawnmower but with a smoother action. Return to the starting position for one rep.

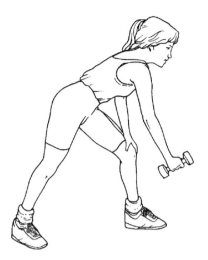

Start position for the bent-over row

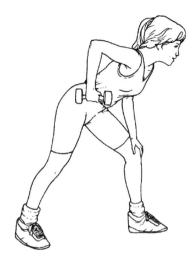

Finish position for the bent-over row

Lower Body Exercises

These exercises target your major lower body muscles. Keep in mind that as a runner, you don't want to overwork your legs, which get a workout every time you run.

Lunges

Stand with feet shoulder-width apart, a dumbbell in each hand in the overhand grip. Step out with your right leg about one stride, landing on your heel and rolling your foot down flat against the floor. Bend both knees so that your right thigh is parallel to the floor (do not let your right knee go beyond your right foot). Your left thigh will be perpendicular to it, and your left heel will lift off the floor. Your arms remain by your sides during the exercise. Return to the starting position by rolling off the ball of your right foot. Alternate legs as you do your reps.

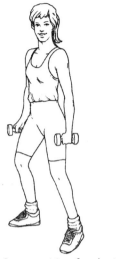

Start position for the Lunge

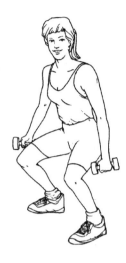

Finish position for the Lunge

Leg Extensions

Choose a chair with firm back support and in which, when you're sitting, your feet rest flat on the floor. Sitting in the chair, put the ankle weights on both feet. One leg at a time, squeeze with your thigh as you lift your leg until your knee is straight. Control the descent. This is 1 rep.

Leg Curls

Lie on the floor, with your arms at your side and the weights around your ankles. Turn your head to one side and lift both feet toward your buttocks, bringing your heels as close to your buttocks as you can. Use your abs to keep your hips pressing into the floor and lower your legs to the starting position for 1 rep.

Exercises for Abs and Back

Use the following exercises to strengthen your abdominal and back muscles. You can do some of these every day, so long as you don't overdo it.

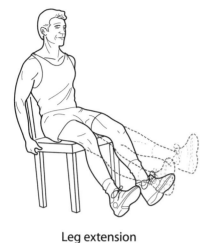

Leg extension

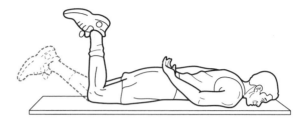

Leg curl

Pelvic Tilt

Lying on your back on the floor, preferably on a mat or folded towel for some cushion, bend your knees, rest your heels on the floor, and let your toes point up. Keep your arms at your side. Imagine gravity pulling your bellybutton onto the floor so that your lower back is flattened against the floor. This will cause your pelvis to rise slightly, and you should feel your abs tighten. Hold this position for several seconds, then relax and repeat. Do 3 sets of 10 reps.

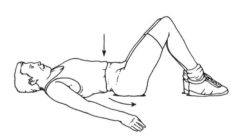

Position for the pelvic tilt

Abdominal Crunch

Lie on your back with your knees bent and feet flat on the floor, about shoulder-width part. Bring your arms up and put your hands under your head, thumbs pointing toward your ears. Don't interlock your fingers, even if your fingers overlap. Keep your head extended from your body so that your

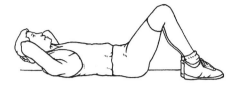

Start for the abdominal crunch

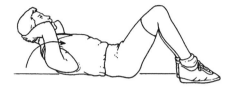

Finish for the abdominal crunch

chin isn't digging into your chest. Start raising your trunk, curling up from your spine, using your abs—not your hands—to pull yourself up.

Keep your elbows to the side and raise yourself up only enough to lift your shoulder blades off the floor. Pause, then bring your trunk back into position slowly for one repetition. Start by doing 3 sets of 15 reps, adjusting according to whether it feels like too much or not enough.

To increase the intensity of your ab crunch workout, try doing your reps with your legs off the floor, crossed at your ankles. Keep your knees bent and your butt on the floor.

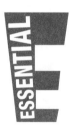

Rather than lifting heavy weights only a few times like bodybuilders and powerlifters do, emphasize lighter weights and more repetitions (12–15). Don't overdo exercises that might leave your legs fatigued for your next run. Instead, concentrate your efforts on your upper body and carefully choose the lower extremity exercises that work for you.

Weight-Training Tips

For a successful weight-training experience, keep the following guidelines in mind:

- Warm up before lifting and stretch thoroughly afterward.
- Run prior to lifting, and avoid weight training leg work on days before races, speed workouts, or long runs.
- Lift every other day or a minimum of 3 days per week.

- Emphasize lighter weights and more repetitions rather than heavy weights for a few reps.
- Don't hold your breath while lifting weights; breathe in on the relaxation phase and out while performing the hard part of the exercise.
- Move your body through the entire range of motion of the exercise, making sure you don't lock your joints while performing the exercise.
- Follow the sequence of legs first, upper body second, and midsection last, remembering to work your abdominal muscles.
- In each sequence, exercise the larger muscle groups first, followed by the smaller groups.

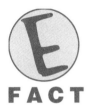

FACT

Remember, you probably won't lose weight as you incorporate a weight-conditioning program in your present training. Instead, you will gain muscle and lower body fat (assuming you eat sensibly). Thus the scale can be very misleading. As you lose fat and gain muscle, your clothes will fit better, and you'll look and feel great!

Run First, Lift Later

Runners should ideally run first and do strength training second, preferably not back-to-back. The best thing to do is schedule several hours between a run and your strength workout. You may run in the morning and then do your strength routine at lunchtime or in the evening. If you are forced to perform the two routines together, do your run first and then your strength training. If you're doing a long run or a speed workout, hold off on the strength training afterward. You'll probably be too tired to perform it properly.

Some have recommended that you perform your hard running and strength training on the same day (but separate the two), followed by an easy run the next day so you have time to recover. Experiment to see what feels right to you. You might find it easier to do your strength training on a light running day or even on a rest day. For more advanced runners, if you do strength training on a rest day, go very easy on the legs or skip the leg workouts entirely if you will be racing or doing a speed work session the next day.

Chapter 8

Building Physical and Mental Strength

Over the past few years, runners of all abilities have discovered the many benefits of cross-training as a means to enhance total conditioning and running performance. They have also found that sharpening their mental state and learning to connect to their bodies helps their overall running performance as well. Yet despite the variety and popularity of cross-training options, some runners still question why they should incorporate activities from cycling to yoga into their training program if running is their primary focus.

8

Cross-Training

Although cross-training provides numerous benefits, too much of a good thing can be counterproductive and detrimental to your running. For example, partaking of certain cross-training activities on a scheduled rest day can leave you tired prior to an important workout, such as a long run (especially if you're in training for a half-marathon or marathon).

Furthermore, engaging in certain cross-training activities can actually increase the likelihood of an injury, particularly during the mileage buildup stage. This, in turn, can prevent you from completing the training necessary to attain your goal of finishing a distance event, from a 5K to a marathon. After learning about which cross-training activities are beneficial for running in this chapter, choose your cross-training activities carefully and schedule those sessions to enhance rather than detract from your running goals.

Benefits and Purposes of Cross-Training

Some of the great benefits of cross-training are that it adds variety to your training and decreases the chance of burnout. Also, certain activities, such as cycling, strengthen running-related muscle groups and soft connective tissue and so help to prevent running injury. You can occasionally substitute cross-training for easy day running as an aerobic workout.

Cross-training, of course, provides an extra way to burn fat. Many cross-training activities, such as rowing or using the Versa Climber, increase upper body strength. Upper body strength is very important in races of all distances, since neck and shoulder muscles often become fatigued. Upper body strength is also important for going uphill.

Precautions and Considerations

Remember, cross-training is not intended to replace running but rather to supplement it. According to the concept of sports specificity, a 90-minute bike ride can't substitute for a 90-minute run. A 90-minute bike ride doesn't provide the training effect needed to run a longer race such as a half-marathon.

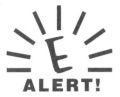
ALERT!

Use common sense when deciding whether to add a particular sport to your fitness regimen. Avoid high-impact fitness routines, especially those with quick or sudden movements. Don't participate strenuously in sports in which quick movements can traumatize the soft connective tissue that surrounds the knees and ankles.

Sudden strains or tears resulting from just a fun pickup game can seriously sideline your running goals, so if you've been putting in training time for a big race, why risk it? Also avoid high-impact sports with quick or sudden movements like tennis, racquetball, basketball, soccer, volleyball, downhill skiing, kick-boxing, and aerobic dance.

Ideal Cross-Training Activities

The following are cross-training activities ideally suited to enhance your running performance. They are recommended because they are all north-south exercises, which place little side-to-side lateral pressures on your body, especially your leg joints, muscles, and connective tissue. Although these cross-training activities offer good cardiovascular workouts, they also give the legs a heavy-duty workout and therefore should not be done on scheduled leg rest days.

Cycling

Cycling exercises some of the same muscle groups as running, such as the quadriceps and shins, both of which don't develop as rapidly from workouts as the calf muscles and hamstrings. Cycling also strengthens the connective tissue of the knee, hip, and ankle regions, thus reducing the risk of injury. After a stressful run, cycling can loosen fatigued leg muscles.

There are three types of biking to try: road riding; mountain biking; and stationary cycling. Taking place on the road, road biking allows you to travel long distances with speed. Mountain bikes are two-wheel, all-terrain vehicles that can be ridden almost anywhere. Although mountain biking is a lot of fun and challenging, its jarring nature makes falls risky. Road and stationary cycling are better alternatives. With stationary cycling, you can workout indoors year-round regardless of inclement weather. Stationary cycling offers the additional benefit of being able to safely listen to music or read while working out.

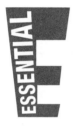

Remember these cycling tips: First, always maintain control when riding your bike. To slow down or stop, feather the brakes, alternating between squeezing and releasing them. Also, be aware of cars. Don't assume that drivers see you. When you ride past parked cars, watch for car doors opening suddenly. Observe traffic signals and signs, and use hand signals to indicate turns or stops.

A few things to keep in mind: Refrain from cycling on a scheduled rest day. Since it's much more difficult to run after cycling, run prior to heading out on your bike. Spin easily, as opposed to grinding big gears. Be sure that your seat height and pedals are properly positioned. Finally, always wear a helmet, and leave the iPod at home!

Water Activities

For the compulsive athlete, swimming is one of the best cross-training activities to add to your running regimen. Swimming gives tired leg muscles a breather while providing an excellent upper body workout. Additionally, water has a therapeutic effect on all muscle groups. Although gentle kicking alleviates some muscle soreness and fatigue, avoid using the kickboard for hard kick sets on your running rest day.

If you swim for the aerobic benefit, do not be concerned that your heart rate does not get as high as during other activities. The loss of gravitational force, the horizontal position, and the cooling effect of the water temperature all contribute toward keeping your heart rate low.

A low heart rate does not mean that your aerobic efforts are in vain. Remember, aerobic exercise is about oxygen utilization, and the heart rate mirrors what is happening on an oxygen level. But in this case, the mirror gives a distorted picture of what's really going on. Even though swimming conditions yield relatively lower heart rate numbers, your body is still processing oxygen, and that's what counts. A general rule is that the swimming heart rate is typically 10–20 beats per minute less than that for dry land activities.

Another type of water cross-training activity is deep water running. In deep water running, you are suspended vertically in a pool by wearing a flotation belt around your waist or torso. Although your feet don't touch the bottom of the pool, you then simulate running.

This cross-training activity is just what the doctor ordered for the rehabilitation of many running injuries. Because there is no shock from footstrike, deep water running is a perfect alternative to a midweek easy day run. The resistance of the water gives you all the benefits of running but none of the shock of footstrike associated with road running. Even though it is possible to run in the water without floatation aids, find a pool that offers these devices (such as vests or belts) for a workout at once easier on your upper body yet more specific in targeting your leg muscles.

Exercise Machines

One popular cross-training machine is the egrometer, or rowing machine. As scullers have known for centuries, rowing is a terrific all-body exercise, strengthening your back, buttocks, and legs and developing your shoulders and arms.

Rowing involves a two-stroke movement referred to as the drive and the recovery, which together produce a smooth and continuous action. It's important to follow good form on a rowing machine, so make sure you ask your health club to show you how to use it properly. This is another highly beneficial activity to do on a rest day. It strengthens the hips, buttocks, and upper body while sparing the legs from heavy pounding.

In addition to rowing machines, you can also try the Nordic Track and other ski-simulator machines. Designed to simulate cross-country skiing, these machines, when used properly, are highly effective in building aerobic conditioning, muscular strength, and endurance. In short, they provide an excellent workout for runners. The dual action movement of both upper and lower body challenges your ability to coordinate two different movements.

One of the most popular machines in the gym these days is the elliptical trainer. Offering a total-body cardiovascular workout, its elliptical motion combines the effects of classic cross-country skiing, stair climbing, and walking without any pounding of the joints. You can program the elliptical trainer to operate in a forward, backward, or combination of motions, providing a low-impact workout for all the major muscles in the legs. The backward motion emphasizes the *gluteal* muscles (buttocks). You can achieve a good upper body workout by using the two poles located on either side of the machine in conjunction with leg motion. Not only is an elliptical training machine versatile, it is fun to use. You can program it to maintain you at your strongest yet safest capacity, you can monitor your heart rate, and you can even customize your workout.

The climbing wall is another piece of equipment that more and more gyms, community centers, and schools are providing. Climbing provides an excellent total-body workout and is mentally and physically challenging, combining balance with footwork and technique. Gyms with indoor climbing walls have the ropes and equipment you need on hand, so you don't have to invest in them. Although it doesn't give a high-intensity cardiovascular workout, it's another way to stretch your muscles while challenging yourself—and can be very entertaining.

Walking

That's right, good old walking is a wonderful way to cross-train. It's an underrated activity with enhanced therapeutic benefits following a long run or speed work. Although walking is not a substitute for an easy running day, a relaxed 2–3 mile stroll is a good way to loosen up your legs the day before a big race. And depending on the type of injury, speed walking is an invaluable rehabilitation activity for maintaining cardiovascular fitness.

Pilates

Pilates was originally called contrology by its founder, Joseph Pilates. Of German and Greek descent, Joseph Pilates emigrated to the United States in the early 1900s and opened a studio in New York City where he and his wife, Clara, taught his particular exercise method. Pilates' concept was to focus on core postural muscles to support the spine for correct alignment, an approach adopted by hospital rehabilitation programs ever since. Recently, Pilates has become very popular with the general public, particularly with those looking for a gentle method of increasing core strength, flexibility, and movement.

Pilates is typically taught in health clubs, where private or semiprivate instruction is available on special Pilates equipment or group mat classes that are conducted without equipment. Pilates uses the resistance of the body to condition and correct itself, with the goal of lengthening and aligning the spine. Like yoga, Pilates offers a low-impact form of strengthening and toning muscles while helping you get more in tune with your body.

Yoga

Increasingly, runners are finding that yoga, in contrast to more strenuous forms of cross-training, provides them with additional strength and flexibility without muscle pounding. Bearing in mind that skeletal muscles work in pairs, what happens during running is that the foot, leg, and hip muscles experience a heavy amount of pounding, tightening, and shortening. Left unattended, these compromised muscles are stressed, possibly leading to injury. Stretching brings them back into balance, keeping them soft and supple so they can do their job.

Since muscles help maintain posture and balance, if these are out of sync, the stressful demands of running will aggravate any preexisting conditions. Many runners simply run in pain and learn to live with it. Yoga can help identify and treat these nagging sources of pain, leading to more enjoyable running—and more years of it.

Turning the Focus Inward

Yoga focuses the mind on the internal movements of the body so that mind, body, and breath are integrated. In an article in *Yoga Journal* on how yoga and running complement each other, Baron Baptiste and Kathleen Finn Mendola write, "In addition to physically counteracting the strains of running, yoga teaches the cultivation of body wisdom and confidence. As you develop a greater understanding of the body and how it works, you become able to listen and respond to messages the body sends you. This is especially important in running, where the body produces a lot of endorphins. These 'feel good' chemicals also double as nature's painkillers, which can mask pain and the onset of injury or illness. Without developed body intuition, it's easier to ignore the body's signals."

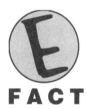

There are different types of yoga, including Hatha, Ashtanga, Iyengar, Vinyasa, and Bikram. It's good to know which type might be best for you before signing up for a class, though you'll find that different people— including instructors—use the terms to mean different things.

Other Benefits

Yoga's focus on breathing can be extremely beneficial to runners. In fact, the *Indian Journal of Medical Research* published a study showing that athletes who practiced yogic breathing (pranayama) were able to exercise more intensely at the same heart rate compared to those who didn't. According to the Pranayama Institute in New Mexico, "The system of pranayama is credited with conferring upon its practitioner a calm, balanced, and focused mind, increased vitality, and longevity."

Suzanne Goldston, a yoga instructor, shared her perspective on *www.marathontraining.com*: "In your yoga practice, you are taught to breath through the nose, keeping the lips together. This allows the nose to do its job. The nose warms, moisturizes and filters the air as well as affecting the nervous system differently than mouth breathing. I'm not suggesting you stop using the mouth to breath[e]. What's important is an increased awareness of the breath, a deepening and steadying of it, and taking the breath deep into the pit of the lungs.

"The richest supply of blood, which is used to transport the breath to the muscles where it becomes energy for you, is in the bottom of the lungs. Because the majority of us are chest breathers, we never really access the entire lungs. As we learn to do this, our lung capacity will increase which will automatically increase our stamina."

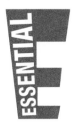

International spiritual leader, artist, and activist Sri Chinmoy says, "The body's capacity and the soul's capacity, the body's speed and the soul's speed, go together. Running and physical fitness help us both in our inner life of aspiration and in our outer life of activity."

Meditation

"Just a minute," you might say. "How does sitting and thinking about nothing benefit my running program?" The benefit of meditation to your running program is in increased focus, just as with yoga. Even if you aren't ready to incorporate yoga into your overall exercise program, perhaps you have time to meditate. If so, you'll notice the benefits of meditation to your running program as well as to other aspects of your life almost immediately. These include:

- Increased blood flow
- Increased brain wave coherence
- Increased self-confidence and feelings of well-being
- Increased exercise tolerance
- Decreased muscle tension
- Decreased blood pressure
- Decreased anxiety, depression, and moodiness

Do some research, and you'll soon discover that meditation can benefit you physically, psychologically, and spiritually. And a better you makes a better runner.

Chapter 9

On the Road All Year

Running is an activity you can do any time of the year. But running intelligently during different seasons requires forethought and specific strategies, especially during the extreme seasons of winter and summer. This chapter gives you the practical and medical information necessary to deal with the elements and enjoy running all year round. If you use common sense, dress correctly, stay hydrated, follow the normal protocol of letting someone know your running route, and not overexert yourself on your training runs, you should be able to stick to a training schedule through all seasons.

Running in Cold Weather

Depending upon your geographic location, winter may not be an optimal time to plan a dramatic increase in mileage or to add speed work to your training regimen. Cold and icy conditions make running more hazardous. Slipping, muscle guarding (a muscle spasm in response to a painful stimulus), and cool muscles can contribute to posterior muscle group and groin pulls.

Cold Weather Strategies

Warm up well before going out, and be especially careful when running on surfaces that are wet or icy. Shorten your stride, and run slower than usual. When running just after a winter storm, if you have a choice of running on ice or snow, choose the snow. You will be less likely to slip because the traction is better.

To help yourself keep warm, a good strategy to remember is to run out against the wind and return with the wind at your back. The greater the amount of cold air passing over your exposed body surface, the faster your body will cool off. By running against the wind, you'll be facing the most environmental stress when you are fresh and running faster. When you are fatigued at the end of a run and expending less energy, you will produce less body heat and your core temperature will have a greater tendency to drop. The wind behind you will help keep you moving.

Dressing for Cold Weather Runs

It is important to protect all areas of your body from exposure. This includes your head, hands, feet, legs, arms, and chest. Also, don't forget your other more delicate parts: Men should consider investing in underwear with an insulated front panel for extra protection.

To protect your feet, which conduct cold through the soles of your running shoes as they strike the cold trails or roads, wear absorbent and dry socks. Polypropylene or acrylic material can wick moisture away, which prevents moisture from forming around your feet while you run and turning to ice when you stop running. You can cover a thin inner sock with a thicker outer sock, provided this doesn't pad your foot so much that you can barely squeeze your foot into your shoe. Immediately following your run, change into a dry pair of socks.

Polypropylene, Varitherm, Skinsense, Cocona, and CoolMax are names of fabrics designed to keep your body either warm and dry or cool and dry. No longer is it necessary to wear multiple layers of T-shirts, sweatshirts, or even a parka to stay warm in the coldest weather. Although you still need to layer, today's materials are less bulky, more comfortable, and better designed to protect against the elements.

A combination to keep you toasty and dry consists of a thin layer of synthetic material to pull moisture away from your body, covered with fleece for insulation, then topped with a breathable, waterproof layer.

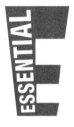

Your skin is the part of your body most exposed to environmental conditions. Nourish and protect it by staying hydrated (whether it's hot or cold out), and wear a sunscreen when you run. Sunblock and moisturizer help prevent a weathered face.

A facemask or scarf further minimizes exposure, especially of the thin skin on your face, and a hat and gloves are musts. For your head, choose a lightweight synthetic fabric that wicks away moisture and won't itch. For hands in relatively mild temperatures, some runners wear painters' gloves as recommended by Bill Rogers. For colder weather, you can wear inner polypropylene gloves with an outer layer of mittens. Choose a soft and absorbent material that can also go in the wash, since cold air hitting the warmer air from your nose will cause your nose to run, in which case wiping it with the back of your hand is the most practical solution.

For your legs, you can add sweatpants over polypropylene tights, or if it is exceptionally cold, wear Gore-tex or nylon pants on the outer layer.

Running in Hot Weather

The best defense against heat is hydration. Therefore, when the temperature goes up, so should your fluid intake. Water should always be your number one drink of choice. Drink before, during, and after you run. Drink before you go to sleep, and drink when you wake up. In short, drink water often throughout the day, regardless of weather conditions. In general, you should drink at least eight glasses of water a day. When it's really hot out, you can easily double this amount.

Always drink before you run, and try to drink about 8 ounces every 25 minutes while you run. Although just water is fine for runs of up to an hour, you will find that sports drinks maintain your performance level for runs over one hour. Most popular sport drinks have a low level of electrolytes and also contain carbohydrates (both simple and more complex polymers) to help speed up glycogen replacement.

Please don't count coffee, beer, or other caffeinated and alcoholic beverages as part of your daily tally of fluids. Although research has shown that caffeine does seem to enhance performance, coffee is a diuretic and a dehydrator. And depending on how long your run is, remember that a caffeine buzz can turn into a wilt. You may not want to skip coffee before you run, but just make sure you drink plenty of water, too.

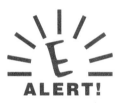
ALERT!

It's important to stay hydrated regardless of the weather or the distance you're running. It's also important to be aware of how much you drink and what you drink during the course of any day. That's because you can also suffer from hyponatremia, or water intoxication. This occurs when fluid intake (including sports drinks) exceeds fluid loss during exercise, resulting in an imbalance between the body's water and sodium levels.

Immediately following exercise, muscles are most receptive to absorbing carbohydrates (which later convert to glycogen in the muscles), which is why you'll often find bagels and PowerBars or other energy bars offered at the end of a race. But don't forget to meet your overall fluid replacement needs with water as well as with fluids containing ample carbohydrates, such as fruit or vegetable juices.

To help you stay hydrated during long, hot summers of running, consider stopping at every water fountain you pass and taking a drink. Don't forget to give yourself a minimum of two weeks to acclimate to the heat. The best way to do this is by running a slow 3–4 miles, making sure you have enough water. Gradually increase your distance and cumulative time running.

Also try combining treadmill running and outside running to get more distance on really hot days. During the first hot, humid days of spring and summer, slowly build your mileage to acclimate to these conditions before considering running at a faster pace. In fact, many seasoned runners put their fast-paced efforts on hold until cooler weather returns. Additionally, try to miss the heat by running early in the morning or late at night. Remember, though, that if you run early in the morning, you may experience more humidity. And, of course, consider using an indoor treadmill on the worst days. That way you can get a workout with a few more miles in a cooler environment.

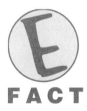

FACT

Perspiration and evaporation of perspiration are the primary means for the body to cool during exercise. Sweat glands become active as body core temperature rises. One liter of sweat is generated during the expenditure of about 500 kilocalorie (kcal). Skin blood flow also increases significantly during exercise. Blood flowing near the surface results in cooling by both conduction and convection.

Heat-Induced Illness

Several illnesses can be induced by heat. The first, heat exhaustion, is caused by dehydration. The symptoms include chills, lightheadedness, dizziness, headache, and nausea. Body temperature usually rises to between 100°–102°F and profuse sweating is evident. To treat heat exhaustion, move to a cool, shaded area, call an ambulance, and drink fluids until help arrives.

Heat stroke, another heat-induced illness, is caused by a sudden failure of the body's thermoregulatory system. Not only is this dangerous, but it can also be fatal. Heat stroke initially presents like heat exhaustion, but can rapidly progress to more serious neurological symptoms, such as disorientation, loss of consciousness, and seizures. Body temperature can rise higher than 104°F. Sweating is often absent, but the skin can be quite moist from earlier perspiration. The pulse of a person afflicted with heat stroke is usually over 160 beats per minute, and blood pressure may be low.

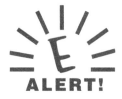

ALERT!

Make sure you are aware of any medical conditions you have or medications you are taking that affect your tolerance for exercise in the heat. Medical conditions affecting heat tolerance include diabetes, high blood pressure, anorexia nervosa, bulimia, obesity, and fever.

If you are suffering from heat stroke, your core temperature must be reduced immediately. Kidney damage (acute nephropathy) occurs in about 35 percent of cases. This is a result of *rhabdomyolysis* (muscle breakdown) and *myoglobulinuria* (excretion of muscle breakdown products), which contribute to kidney injury. Liver damage is also evident when liver enzymes are measured following heatstroke. Oftentimes getting packed in ice reduces core temperature. If you suspect you are suffering from heat stroke, it is vital that you get medical attention.

Avoiding Heat Stress Injury

To avoid heat exhaustion or heat stroke, drink plenty of fluids (preferably water) 25–30 minutes before exercise and then 8 ounces every 25–30 minutes while exercising. After exercising, drink more fluids than you think you need, especially if you are over the age of forty. Don't wait until you feel thirsty; by that time you're already dehydrated. Drinking fluids while you exercise as well as when you're finished helps speed your recovery.

You can also protect yourself from the heat by gradually building up your tolerance for running in warmer weather. Stay fit, and don't overestimate your level of fitness. Individuals with a higher VO_2 max (how much oxygen your body can transport to your muscles every minute) are more tolerant of heat than those with a lower level.

Dressing Cool for the Heat

Even if you feel like you don't want to wear anything at all when it's really hot out, don't make that mistake! The worst thing to do is to overheat your body and then, with no protection, expose it to rapid cooling. This can cause lightheadedness and dizziness.

When running in the heat, wear lightweight fabrics that wick away moisture, support your body, and neutralize odor. There are all sorts of comfortable and fashionable shorts and tops available for men and women. Workout apparel these days is about comfort, fit, performance, and style—no more baggy cotton T-shirts and gym shorts for enthusiasts who value comfort and protection.

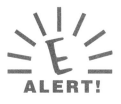

If you run when it's dark (at any time of the year), wear a reflective garment. Reflective garments are made of high-tech materials that provide safety, comfort, and temperature control to keep you cool in the summer and warm in the winter.

As for upper body wear, women can opt for a colorful sports bra and men a breezy fabric singlet. Thin, absorbent socks can keep your feet from getting too sweaty. To keep sweat from dripping into your eyes, you might want to wear a headband or a visor. Even though baseball caps shield the sun, they trap heat—something to consider on hot, humid days. Don't forget to apply heavy-duty sunscreen, especially on your face.

Running Indoors

Running outside in inclement weather prepares you for races, which don't stop for the weather (save, of course, for extreme weather like thunderstorms, hurricanes, and snow storms). Running outside regardless of the weather is a healthy and invigorating experience.

Even so, running indoors is reliable, convenient, limits your exposure to outside risks, and can be more sociable if you choose. If there's a school or college near you that has an indoor track you can use, consider doing so. It's a nice alternative to running on a treadmill at home or at the gym. Be careful, though, as some indoor tracks are shorter than ⅛ of a mile. Short tracks have more turns, which can adversely affect your knees, ankles, and hips. Look for tracks that are longer than at least ⅛ mile in length, and check whether it's permissible to change directions halfway through your run, which is better for your legs. Some tracks prefer that everyone run in the same direction.

A treadmill is a good option for indoor running and can be done at home, at a gym, or club. There are new indoor treadmills coming to market all the time. The best indoor treadmill is the one that works for you. Experiment with several before you hone in on one, and be receptive to trying new ones that show up in your gym.

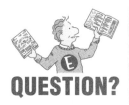

QUESTION?

How do I know my miles per hour?
Pace is the number of minutes it takes to travel 1 mile. To determine your pace, divide 60 by your speed in miles per hour. For example: If your treadmill speed equals 3.5 mph, divide 60 by 3.5. You are running a 17-minute mile.

Running on treadmills is recommended when you have no choice and you don't want to miss a workout. The treadmill's convenience is wonderful, but ultimately it will not help you train for long-distance running. Those in training for a marathon still need to do a large percentage of running on roads, particularly with those all-important long runs. As you run indoors, remember to focus on your form. When you exercise, proper posture and technique are essential to maximizing your effort and avoiding injury. Many runners respect the importance of posture and mechanics when doing outside sports but give little thought to these when exercising indoors on equipment.

Using the Treadmill

Most commercial equipment in health clubs is clearly labeled with instructions. But if you are still unclear about how to use the equipment, ask the staff for assistance. If you are going to buy a piece of equipment, make sure you get a demonstration on how to properly use and maintain it (along with a warranty and instruction manual if buying from a retail store).

Here are some tips for using a treadmill:

- Learn how to use it before you use it.
- Use manual mode for complete control of the intensity (speed, elevation, and resistances).
- Pay attention to your intensity level and your use of distractions to pass the time (music, reading, talking, thinking) so you don't overdo it.
- Drink water during exercise to stay hydrated.
- Use a fan to keep from getting overheated.

Once you get used to the feeling of the ground moving beneath your feet, you will truly appreciate running on a treadmill. The treadmill is obedient and will keep the speed and elevation steady at the levels you set. The speed and elevation settings determine the treadmill's intensity. You can either control the settings yourself through manual mode or experiment with preprogrammed workouts. Many home models allow you to program your own workouts and keep them in memory as a preprogrammed workout.

Learn how to control your treadmill:

- Know where the stop button is located.
- Practice grabbing the handrail and standing on the nonmoving side panels before stopping the machine.
- Stay focused and avoid turning your body or looking directly down at your feet.
- Keep children and pets away from the treadmill and from the operating key.

- Position the back of the treadmill away from a wall so that you do not bump into it.

Shopping for a Treadmill

Commercial treadmills can accommodate persons of most body weights; home models are typically built to withstand body weights not greater than 250 pounds. If you presently walk and are planning to eventually run on the treadmill, a minimum horsepower of 1.5–2.0 is recommended. Be sure to ask the salesperson whether the machine has elevation change capability. Elevation capability gives you more variety in the type of workouts you can do (or progress to doing).

Noise is difficult to detect on a showroom floor, but listen for it anyway. Compare the store surroundings with those where you will put your machine. If it seems a bit noisy in the showroom and you plan to put the treadmill in a small room with little insulation, expect that it will be even louder at home.

Take measurements to make sure you have enough room for the treadmill you are considering, and for safety purposes, avoid positioning the treadmill with its back close to a wall. One small misstep and you could be thrown with an unplanned back injury—as well as finding yourself in need of some home remodeling.

Safety Features

You absolutely want an emergency pull/stop mechanism. In the event you unexpectedly fall (or move more than a few feet from the treadmill), a light emergency cord connected to the treadmill control panel would disengage and instantly stop the motor. Some people prefer to wear this chord clipped onto their clothing; others prefer that it rest within reach on top of the treadmill. Either way, this mechanism is an effective and valuable safety feature.

Another safety feature preferred by many people is a treadmill railing. Front rails are best; side rails are steadying but for some can get in the way during exercise. If you aren't sure which you prefer, this is another reason to check out several treadmills and feel the differences between models.

Deck, Speed, and Other Features

Deck flexibility makes a difference in how your bones and joints feel in response to the treadmill's impact. There is no standard word to describe how flexible the deck is, but you need to inquire whether the treadmill you are considering has such a system. Good treadmills have some type of flexible deck system.

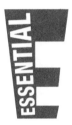

Do not waste your money on nonelectrical or human-powered treadmills. The movement of the belt is stiff, sluggish, and uneven, which doesn't feel like something you'd want to stay on for more than a minute. The mental and physical energy spent on this kind of treadmill is better spent on one more enjoyable and easier to use.

You also want a smooth belt action, which means that the machine can pull its own weight (and yours) without hesitation or knocking. Ask what the maximum speed and maximum elevation of the machine are. If you consistently run a blazing 6-minute mile or faster, some treadmills cannot match your speed, and therefore you would not want to buy them.

The components panel displays such measurements as your distance, speed, calories burned, elevation, and heart rate, as well as your programmable workouts. The more components you want to see displayed on the console, the higher the price. But do not let that discourage you. Envision yourself walking and running on the treadmill for years to come and think about how much enjoyment and motivation you will derive from knowing how you perform in those seemingly trivial areas that the console displays.

Finally, note which creature comforts (if any) are important to you, such as cup and magazine holders. Make a list of questions and bring it with you when shopping so all your concerns are addressed before buying.

Chapter 10

On the Road to Speed and Distance

How can you increase your speed? Most runners ask this question once they become more accomplished. Indeed, one of the best things about running is being able to compete not only against others but also against yourself. Improvement is almost always possible, but it is also dependent upon so many factors, including one's age, current fitness level, genetics, experience level, type of training program, etc. If you run faster this week, can you run even faster next? Runners have been asking this question since the Greeks staged the first Olympics. This chapter gives you insight into adding speed work to your workout.

Adding Speed Work

Incorporating some carefully designed faster-paced runs is essential to a program seeking faster performance in your daily training runs and in races you enter. However, the key point to remember is that speed work is an advanced training technique for an experienced runner and not for a true beginner.

For the more accomplished runner, though, incorporating some advanced running techniques is necessary to improve your time from one race to the next. Your best race times are referred to as PRs (personal records) or PBs (personal bests).

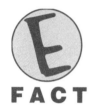

FACT

PR (personal record) and PB (personal best) both represent your fastest time posted at a given distance. In order to claim a PR or PB, you must perform on a track or a road race course certified as accurate by USA Track and Field (USATF), the national governing body for track and field, long-distance running, and race walking.

In short, don't entertain the notion of adding speed work to your training regimen until you have been running regularly (logging 20–25 miles per week) for a minimum of a year. Doing so without this solid mileage base greatly increases your chance of incurring an injury. If you do decide to focus on this aspect of your running, it is important to read this entire section before beginning any speed workout on your own.

The Risks

Despite the benefit of increasing your speed, incorporating advanced training techniques exponentially increases your risk of injury. You really need to think about whether you are willing, after months of training, to risk injury that prevents you from participating in your chosen event.

Even runners who feel ready to work on improving their speed need to be careful. Speed workouts are sessions in which you need to push yourself.

But pushing too hard may result in injury. You have to be smart. Exert yourself—for there is no gain without some physical discomfort—but don't be macho. A mistake here can result in serious, if not languorous, injuries that can keep you from running for weeks or even months at a time.

The Benefits

There are many benefits to adding advanced running techniques to your training beyond merely improving your speed and chocking up faster race times. The physical gains attained through speed work are more numerous than you might think. There's the obvious, which of course is improved strength and speed. However, these are actually byproducts of the training. With higher intensity training, you now have a better oxygen delivery system. You can run faster and still stay at a comfortable, aerobic (meaning, using air) pace. Your body becomes more efficient at delivering oxygen to your muscles, and your muscles function better while using less oxygen.

When your body exceeds its capacity to use oxygen as fuel, you begin using glycogen as your primary fuel source. A byproduct of this anaerobic (without oxygen) method of energy production is lactic acid.

Rather than your body going into oxygen debt (characterized by that heavy, burning feeling in your legs), in which your muscles tie up due to a buildup of lactic acid from a lack of oxygen, your anaerobic system can be trained as was your cardiovascular system. With specific anaerobic training, you can exceed limits that previously held you back.

Fine-Tuning Your Mechanics

If you train diligently, your running mechanics will surely improve, especially if you've been able to implement the recommendations of a running coach or experienced runners. Your arm drive, stride, and breathing will all improve as a result of incorporating advanced running techniques into your training. You will run faster with less effort during your daily runs, and your speed will improve for races you wish to enter.

Mental Edge

The mental benefits of doing speed work result from your setting and achieving time-related goals. Running PRs off your improved speed is quite fulfilling and can be highly motivating. Speed work can be challenging and sometimes quite uncomfortable, perhaps even painful (not to be confused with the pain associated with injury, however).

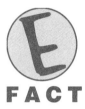

FACT

You can usually find a competent coach through a running club, a specialty running store, a college or university, or on the Web. Before you commit to a particular coach, ask lots of questions about the coach's background and training philosophy. Be sure that the one you choose is the right one for you.

You are asking your body to perform faster and outside of the aerobic zone, which through training has become comfortable with long, slow runs. You're pushing the limits of your body and mind, past previous physical and mental barriers. The end result is that your mental toughness improves significantly, both during fast-paced training runs and when competing in races of all distances.

Race Strategy

Last, but certainly not least, you'll benefit from planning and implementing a smart race day strategy. Speed workouts furnish you with improved stamina throughout an entire race, which alone results in a better finish time. A smart race strategy entails planning your race in advance. Rather than sprinting through the first part of a 5K (as if you're competing in the Olympic 100-meter finals) and having little energy left for the rest of the race, your experience from running intervals on a track can give you a good idea of what pace you should run during a race.

Quick Guidelines for Speed Work

Some basic guidelines for speed work are as follows:

First, you should be consistently running a minimum of 20–25 miles per week for a year before you even begin to think about including advanced training techniques in your training schedule. If you've never included speed work as part of your training, learn as much as you can from credible sources (books, magazine articles, Web sites) so that you have the knowledge you need to train smart. It is important to confirm that this information is accurate, up-to-date, and from reliable sources.

Be sure to follow the hard-easy method of training if you intend to integrate speed training into your program. For example, do not schedule a speed work session the day after a long run or after participating in a road race. If their longest run of the week is on Sunday, most experienced runners do their speed training during the middle of the week following either an easy run or a complete leg rest day.

If you choose to participate in speed work with a group, be sure to run at a pace appropriate for your ability level. Trying to perform a workout designed for someone else (in particular, for a runner who is significantly faster than you are) greatly increases your chance of incurring an injury and can also be discouraging. To avoid injury, proper warm-ups and cool-downs are essential. These include light jogging followed by stretching both before and after the workout.

No more than 15–20 percent of your total weekly mileage should be fast-paced running. This percentage covers both speed workouts as well as races. You should not increase the volume of your fast-paced running by more than 800 meters per week.

If you elect to do speed workouts during the summer months, schedule them for the early morning or evening to avoid the hottest and most humid times of the day. Pushing the pace in such conditions increases your chance of succumbing to heat illness.

Finally, be careful of what you eat and how late you time your meal or snack before fast-paced running. Experimenting with a variety of food and drink is the best way to determine what your system can tolerate. Don't eat a big lunch if you're planning on doing a fast-paced run later in the afternoon. Instead, have small snacks throughout the day.

Overview of Advanced Training

Speed work can be uncomfortable and, yes, sometimes even painful. But by doing speed workouts, you become accustomed to running faster and tolerating both the physical and mental discomforts when racing. You will also be able to run faster without any extra effort during your easy training runs due to your improved cardiovascular conditioning.

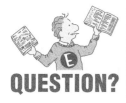

QUESTION?

What are the benefits of doing speed work with a group?
"Doing speed work in a group helps you push yourself. It gives you a sense of competition. It also gives people more inspiration. People feel better in groups. They are more apt to push themselves as they see other people pushing themselves. Misery loves company."—Pam Spadola, Howell, NJ, speed work group leader, Freehold Area Running Club

Through speed work, you can improve your body's ability to run faster with limited oxygen stores available. Additionally, your speed will improve on your easier runs. Like with any training, you need to apply stress in small, progressive steps over a period of weeks. Just as weightlifters work up to lifting a new weight slowly and swimmers increase their ability to hold their breath, runners must gradually adapt their bodies to the stress of running fast in order to improve their tolerance to lactic acid buildup. This is the purpose of speed work.

The Physiological Aspects of Speed Training

Everyone knows that when you sprint or climb a few flights of stairs you get a burning sensation in your legs. This occurs due to your muscles working while being deprived of oxygen. During everyday activities as well as long, slow running, your body uses mostly oxygen as fuel (aerobic running). As you increase the workload on your muscles, your body begins burning stored fuel, called glycogen, for energy. This anaerobic (without oxygen) workout results in an accumulation of lactic acid, which is a byproduct of anaerobic metabolism. With continued effortful movement, this lactic acid accumulates to the point where it begins shutting down your muscles.

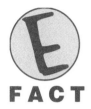

FACT

The point at which your body reaches its maximum capacity for using oxygen and then switches over to accumulating lactic acid is termed the *anaerobic threshold*. With proper speed training, you can raise this threshold, which allows you to run at a faster pace before reaching the point where lactic acid accumulation begins slowing you down.

Another important factor that relates to running performance is your aerobic capacity. This value, also known as your max VO_2, or maximal oxygen uptake, is a measure of how well your body uses large volumes of oxygen during your peak performances. An apparatus used in human performance labs measures your max VO2 while you run all out on a treadmill.

Other inherited qualities can either work for or against you. Your morphology (body type), the ratio of your fast twitch to slow twitch muscle fibers (those who excel at sprinting have higher ratios of fast twitch muscle fibers, in contrast with those who perform better in endurance events who have a higher ratio of slow twitch muscle fibers), and the quality of your cardiorespiratory system all play roles in how well you are able to reach your full potential as a runner. Like your aerobic capacity and anaerobic threshold, most genetic attributes can be minimized or enhanced through proper training.

One of the best ways to do speed work with others is to contact a local running club. You can find a running club by contacting the Road Runners Club of America (*www.rrca.org*) for a list of running clubs throughout the nation. Many running clubs hold weekly speed workout sessions at a local track and sometimes offer seminars at club meetings.

When Do I Begin My Speed Work?

If you want to train seriously for a race, don't start too early or too late. You should train intensely for only three to four months at a time. Additionally, you can usually peak (race your best) only two or three times a year. Over-doing speed work week after week leads to excessive fatigue and burnout. To establish a baseline for determining your present race pace, enter a 5K or 10K race. Then begin your prime-time training three to four months prior to the race at which you want to achieve your best performance.

Where to Run a Speed Workout

The best place to do speed work is at a local outdoor track. You can find a track at a local park, high school, or college. It is worth your while to travel the distance to one of these facilities to do your speed work.

Why do you need to use a real track? You should seek out an existing track because the heart of speed workouts consists of short distance segments from 200–1,600 meters. Tracks are accurately measured so you know exactly how far you are running as well as your exact pace.

Although not essential, the best track to use is one with a synthetic or rubberized surface. Unlike a cinder or asphalt track, the softer surface of a synthetic track is easier on your legs. Oftentimes the surface of a dirt or cinder track is not consistently smooth, which increases the risk of foot and ankle injuries. Running speed work on dirt and cinder surfaces also adds a few seconds to your lap times.

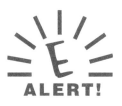

A word about indoor tracks: You have to run several more laps to the mile indoors compared to 4 times around an outdoor track. The turns on indoor tracks are also much tighter than outdoor tracks, which, if you aren't used to this, can wreak havoc on your knees. On the other hand, in the winter an indoor track is a safe, dry haven for dodging the elements.

If you can't get to a track, find a safe place to lay out a running loop for yourself. Try using a bicycle with a cyclo-computer rather than a car odometer to measure your route. There are also new pedometer-like products on the market that measure both your pace and distance covered. A sensor chip attached to the running shoe relays highly accurate pace-distance information to an accompanying watch.

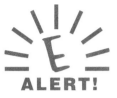

Beginners and novice runners should not run more than one speed-work session a week. In speed work, over time you are incrementally stressing your anaerobic and cardiovascular systems.

Because you will be running short-distance segments such as 200, 400, and 800 meters, you want the mileage marked out to be as accurate as possible. Mileage estimated from a car odometer is inaccurate, making your times less meaningful. You expend both physical effort and mental energy when doing speed work. Therefore, avoid streets with heavy traffic and paths full of bikes and pedestrians—obstacles and distractions that steal the mental focus needed for high-intensity workouts.

Chapter 11

Advanced Running Workouts

A wide variety of workouts encompass advanced training techniques. The most common workouts include hill repeats, fartlek runs, striders (also called pickups), tempo runs, and even road races. Integrated carefully into your training, such workouts make you a stronger and faster runner. Whereas speed workouts should be limited to those with a solid base of running, beginners can incorporate some of the techniques discussed in this chapter. Although all runners need to acknowledge their limitations so they don't push themselves too hard, too soon, incorporating a challenge keeps your running program from becoming too routine.

Hill Repeats

As the name suggests, hill repeats are repetitive charges—running fast-paced efforts up hills. Integrate hill repeats (considered a strengthening workout) into your training schedule immediately after the base-building stage. This will be the time period when you slowly and carefully build weekly mileage levels (with increases no more than 10 percent per week).

Physical Benefits of Hill Repeats

Even if you live in an area with no hills, you can still do hill repeats by finding a highway overpass or bridge with about a 5 percent grade. You generally run hill repeats once a week for three to four weeks to improve your leg strength and as a very important injury prevention measure. Hill repeats are also an excellent means to prepare your cardiovascular system for speed workouts to follow.

Mental Benefits of Hill Repeats

Besides deriving benefits from strengthening your legs, hill repeats enhance your mental toughness for workouts and races on hilly terrain. Although you may never gain an unconditional love for hill training or racing on hilly courses, you will at least face challenging terrains with confidence.

How do you do hill repeats? After a warm-up jog of 1–1½ miles (or a minimum of 12 minutes of easy running), assault the hill at 5K effort pace (that's effort, not speed). The idea is to run up the hill as hard as you can while maintaining good running form.

As you reach the end point of the uphill section (generally 100 meters for the novice and up to 200 meters for the experienced runner), your breathing should feel very labored and your legs quite heavy. Turn around and jog (or walk) very easily down the hill, then continue on flat ground for 30 meters or so before turning around for the next repeat.

Depending on your level of experience, the number of repeats will vary. The novice should do no more than 4 repeats the first week, adding 2 additional repeats each week for the next three to four weeks. The experienced runner can begin with 6 repeats and proceed from there. As with any workout, it is important to cool down by jogging at least a mile (or a minimum of 10–12 minutes).

Hill Repeat Basics:

- Shorten your stride
- Lean slightly into the hill
- Keep your head up, focusing on what's just in front of you rather than the top of the hill or incline
- Maintain a consistent effort up the hill
- Swing your arms (up and down rather than side to side)
- Stay mentally focused and self-directed, pushing forward until you complete the hill repeat

Fartlek Workouts

Fartlek, a Swedish word meaning "speed play," is an unstructured type of speed work that can be quite spontaneous in nature. Like hill repeats, the fartlek workout is considered a transition type of workout that you incorporate into your running training program prior to beginning structured speed training. The central purpose of fartlek runs is to prepare you for the anaerobic demands that more structured speed workouts and racing provide. In short, the fartlek workout is designed to be a fun and easy way to introduce speed training into your program.

Whereas more structured speed workouts, generally done on a track or an accurately measured course, encompass specified periods and distances of fast-paced running followed by recovery periods, the fartlek workout is quite different. You can run a fartlek workout at a fast pace in varying distances and durations.

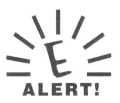
ALERT!

Just as you can run fartlek workouts in a variety of ways, you can perform them on various terrain, including on roads and trails. Before doing fartleks on hilly courses, however, it's best to accustom yourself to these workouts by running them on flat ground.

Fartlek Running Guidelines

Even though it is considered an unstructured workout, there are basic guidelines for fartlek running. Begin your workout with a minimum of 1–1½ miles of easy running (or a minimum of 12 minutes). End with a 1-mile cooldown, throw in speed bursts of varying times and distances, then follow each with a recovery jog.

The idea here is to practice running at a brisk effort (generally faster than your present 5K race pace), employing good running form and training your body to run anaerobically (meaning without oxygen). Push yourself until your breathing becomes labored and your pace begins to drop off. Rather than continuing to push yourself past this point (when you are running at a slow pace with deteriorating form due to fatigue), it's much more beneficial to run fast for a shorter period of time and then to resume when you recover (that is, catch your breath).

Planning a Fartlek Workout

In a fartlek workout, some runners run at a fast pace (at or faster than their current 5K race pace) to a designated landmark such as a telephone pole, then slow down to catch their breath (recover) until they reach the next telephone pole, where they pick up the pace again. They repeat this pattern of running from landmark to landmark until the conclusion of the workout.

Other runners plan their fartlek workout to be more specific. For example, after their warm-up period, they run fast for one minute followed by running a minute at an easy pace to recover. You could repeat this process through the conclusion of the workout, increasing and decreasing the duration and/or distance of fast-paced running at any time. The choice is up to you, based on your perceived level of effort and the amount of discomfort you are willing to experience.

So as not to overdo exercise and risk incurring an overuse injury, you should develop a specific plan for incorporating fartlek workouts into your training program. For example, you might want to run 30 seconds fast followed by 30 seconds easy. Then you could throw in a 45 second burst followed by a 45 second recovery job, and so forth.

The first week the novice might aim for 4 minutes of total fast-paced running (for example, 30 seconds + 30 seconds + 30 seconds + 45 seconds + 45 seconds + 30 seconds + 30 seconds), adding 2 minutes of fast effort for each of the next three weeks. By having a specific plan ahead of time for enduring a cumulation of fast periods of running, you are much less likely to become injured by overdoing your workout.

Striders, Tempo Runs, and Races

Also known as pickups, striders are generally done following your warm-up jog prior to the beginning of an interval session or a road race to prepare your legs and cardiovascular system for the fast-paced running to immediately follow. Like a race car driver revving up the engine prior to the beginning of the Daytona 500, striders get your oxygen and blood flowing at an increased rate so you can perform optimally.

The distance of striders is approximately 80 meters in length. These are best run on a straightaway rather than around curves. Begin by gradually increasing your pace so that you're running with a full stride (but not at full speed) by the 30–40 meters mark. Hold the pace for the next 10 meters before gradually reducing your speed to a jog by the end of the 80 meters.

The purpose of the strider is to achieve a long, full-stride length at a comfortable speed. You do not want to sprint all out in a strider. Turn around and repeat this process 4 times (for a beginner) to 10 times (for an advanced competitor). Time your striders so that your speed workout or race follows a couple of minutes later.

Tempo Runs

The primary purpose of including tempo runs in your regimen is to increase your anaerobic threshold to maintain a faster pace over longer periods of time. The pace of the tempo run should be about 10–15 seconds slower than your present 10K race pace. Depending upon your race goals, the tempo segment of your run can be anywhere from 6–20 minutes or more. When training for longer races such as half-marathons and marathons, you can perform tempo runs of 30 minutes or even longer, running the fast-paced segments at approximately your goal race pace.

Rather than doing a structured warm-up that includes stretching and striders, start out your tempo workout by running easily for at least 12 minutes or longer before cruising into the fast segment. An example of a tempo run workout is to run 12 minutes at tempo pace followed by a 6-minute recovery jog. You could then tack on another 12-minute segment at tempo pace before concluding the balance of your workout with easy running.

Races

Besides being a fun way to run at a faster pace, incorporating races into your long-term training program provides several other benefits. Races are a good way to measure your progress and improvement. Races also allow a beginner to step up from a mileage buildup phase to learning to run a bit faster. The novice and experienced runner can both use early to midseason races as tempo workouts.

Regardless of your rationale for including races as part of your training program, it is important to schedule your races based on the following tenet: Prior to running your next race, allow a day of no racing for each mile you race. For example, if you are running a 10K (6.2 miles), don't run another 10K race for at least seven days afterward. You could, however, run a 5K race the following weekend. Similarly, if you run a half-marathon (13.1 miles), don't run another race of any distance for the following fourteen days. Of course, you need to listen to your body when it comes to running speed workouts within a few days of a race. If your legs feel shot, rest them with easier runs until they feel fresh enough for a hard workout.

Interval Workouts

Interval workouts consist of a series of short, fast-paced runs, generally a mile or less in distance, interspersed with recovery jogs. There are many variations of interval workouts, each with its own rationale but all with a goal of improving overall speed in race distances, from the mile to the marathon.

Prior to beginning any type of interval session, it is very important to begin your workout with a thorough warm-up featuring easy jogging, stretching, and striders. Equally important is the cool-down that concludes the workout.

While repeat interval workouts are most often run on a 400-meter track (commonly found on high school and college campuses), they can also be run elsewhere, such as on roads and trails. However, should you choose to do these on a course other than a track, you need to measure the route accurately (to the exact meter) so that the workout is meaningful.

There are three basic types of interval workouts: repeat intervals, pyramids, and ladders. Each is described below. First, though, some general concepts about intervals need introduction.

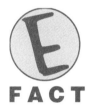

FACT

Interval workouts feature two major components. First, they have a fast-paced segment, called the *repeat,* which is run over a specified distance at a targeted goal time. That is followed by a brief rest period called the *recovery.*

The theory behind the interval workout is simple. Let's use a 5K (3.1 mile) race as an example. Rather than working on improving your speed over the entire 5K distance, it is more effective to run a bit faster than your present race pace over distances shorter than the 5K. Follow these speed intervals with brief periods of rest.

First, you determine your present mile pace in a short distance race such as a 5K. There are several variables in an interval workout that you can tweak to change the level of difficulty. You can adjust the target time for the interval up or down, increase or decrease the recovery (time or distance), and increase or decrease the number of repeats. If you are a novice, an experienced runner or a coach can assist you in designing interval workouts appropriate for both your present ability level and your short- and long-term running goals.

The target time for the interval (the fast-paced segment) is usually based on your current race pace in a short-race distance such as a 5K. The most common interval distances for which to practice fast-pace efforts include 200 meters, 400 meters, 800 meters, 1,200 meters, 1,600 meters, and 1 mile. Although novices first attempting interval workouts might practice running the shorter segments at their current race pace, more experienced competitors would do these 20–30 seconds per mile faster.

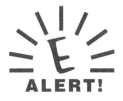

The quality of your interval workout is affected by leg fatigue resulting from not getting enough rest or not warming up properly. You might require a longer warm-up jog or need to stretch a bit more. Environmental conditions such as warm temperatures and high humidity or stiff headwinds also can negatively affect your performance during these fast-paced workouts.

For the experienced runner, the recovery jog following the repeat is typically half the distance of the interval you run. The novice first attempting these workouts should allow a longer recovery period. The recovery period is expressed as a time approximately the same duration as the fast segment previously run.

Repeat Intervals

These are workouts in which the distance of the fast-paced segment remains constant. For example, the workout could feature 6 400-meter repeats with a 200-meter recovery jog after each. Or 4 800-meter repeats each followed by a 400-meter recovery jog is another type of workout.

It is important to run consistent times for the repeats. You should try to run the final repeat in approximately the same time as you ran the first. The idea here is to leave the track feeling that, if you wanted to, you could do 1 or 2 more intervals.

If you find that your speed really falls off after the first couple of intervals, your target time for these may be too fast for your current level of conditioning. You can either adjust the workout from the original plan by increasing your goal times for the repeats (running the repeats at a slower pace), allow yourself more recovery between the fast-paced segments, or bag the workout entirely and attempt it another day.

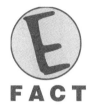

FACT

Abbreviations are often used in books, magazine articles, or by coaches to describe specific speed workouts. For example: 6 × 400M in 1:40, 200R means that you will be asked to run 6 400-meter repeats (once around the track) in 1 minute and 40 seconds, followed by a 200-meter recovery jog after each of the repeats.

Pyramids and Ladders

Pyramids and ladders are also considered part of the interval family. Rather than running the same distances for all your intervals, you vary the length of each interval, running longer or shorter intervals throughout the workout. Pyramid workouts feature fast segments increasing and then decreasing in distance. For example, your fast segments could progress upward from 200–400 meters and topping out at 800 meters before going down again to 400 and then 200 meters.

A ladder is a progression either up or down in interval length. For example, your intervals could progress upward with longer and longer lengths: 200 meters, followed by 400, 800, 1,200, and ending with 1,600 meters. Or you could run the ladder workout in reverse order beginning with the longest distance of your fast-paced segments (1,600, 1,200, 800, 400, 200).

Important Warm-Up and Cool-Down Procedures

With the exception of fartlek and tempo runs (during which you will be doing some easy jogging prior to rolling into their fast-paced segments), it is important to develop a regular, thorough warm-up routine you can use for every interval workout and race. The warm-up is important for three reasons. First of all, running at a fast pace without a proper warm-up greatly increases your chance of incurring an injury. Second, your muscles perform more efficiently and optimally after being properly warmed up. Third, following a consistent routine decreases the high anxiety and stress levels that sometimes precede difficult workouts and races.

Your Warm-Up Routine

It is very important to plan for and allow adequate time for your warm-up so that you're not rushed getting to the starting line of a race. Similarly, you don't want to rush through a warm-up (or a cool-down, for that matter).

Begin your warm-up with a minimum of 12 minutes of easy jogging. When you are racing shorter distances (such as the 5K) or when the weather is cold, you may want to increase the time or distance of your warm-up jog.

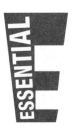

Rather than running lap after lap on a track (which can be quite boring!), do your warm-up on a road or a grass field. Spare your knees, ankles, and hips unnecessary wear and tear resulting from frequent turns on a track.

Next, you want to stretch all your major leg muscles (calves, hamstrings, quads, hips) thoroughly for several minutes. Again, don't rush yourself! While stretching, take a few swigs of water to top off your reservoir. It's better to hydrate at this time so as to have an effective speed workout without interruption. If it's a warm day, however, use common sense and drink fluids as often as conditions dictate.

The last event prior to your speed workout or race is to run 4–10 striders of 80 meters, as described earlier. After completing these, take a minute or two to catch your breath. You are now prepared to run hard.

Your Cool-Down Routine

Don't consider your workout or race over until you cool down properly. Even when performing your daily runs at a comfortable pace, you should finish up a workout by jogging easily the last 10 minutes and then stretch immediately afterward.

After running at a fast pace, it is even more important to jog easily for ten minutes or longer so that your breathing and heart rate can return to normal. Following your cool-down jog, invest 10–15 minutes in stretching your major leg muscles (along with any upper body parts that feel tight) thoroughly before calling it quits. By cooling down properly, your muscles recover effectively from hard workout or race demands. Compared with the runner who rushes through or skips his cool-down, you will find that your muscles feel much less stiff, sore, and fatigued later in the day. In addition, you will be fully recovered and ready to perform optimally for your next workout.

Speed-Work Programs Based on Experience

When developing a program integrating advanced training techniques, it is important to remember that there is no one-size-fits-all approach. Programs must be individualized to meet your present ability level as well as your goals and needs. This section provides a wide range of essential guidelines, both for the runner first attempting speed work and for the accomplished runner.

The Beginner

The beginner is the person who has just started a running program over the past year. As emphasized previously, the beginner's primary focus is to build a base consistently for a year of running 20–25 miles per week. By exercising patience during this time, you will strengthen your leg muscles to later handle the rigors of more advanced training. A beginner pushing the limits by doing speed workouts before leg muscles have strengthened adequately greatly increases the risk of injury.

Rather than including advanced training techniques in their program, it's perfectly fine for beginners to enter distance races of 5K and 10K once a month or so for fun and that way gain experience from running in an organized and competitive forum. By occasionally participating in road races, beginners gather an understanding of their present ability level (race pace) while learning the value of even pacing.

The Novice

A novice runner is one who has consistently been running 20–25 miles per week for a year or more. After this base-building phase, novices can add some advanced training techniques in their training schedule.

This next phase can begin by performing four weeks of hill repeats one time per week. Novices can start with four repeats up a 5 percent grade of 100 meters long, adding two repeats for each of the next three weeks. (Refer to the hill repeat section presented earlier in this chapter for guidelines.)

You can then engage in fartlek runs during the next four weeks as a transition from the hill repeat phase to interval training. The novice should begin with 4 minutes of cumulative fast-paced efforts one time per week and increase the duration by 2 minutes each week for the next three weeks. (Please refer to the fartlek section presented earlier in this chapter for additional guidelines.)

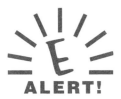
ALERT!

If you are a beginner attempting speed work for the first time, do not jump ahead and attempt workouts designed for an experienced runner. Injury is almost guaranteed! Progress comes with consistent training over months and years. Train only at your present ability level!

Following eight combined weeks of hill and fartlek workouts, novices are now ready to include more structured speed work in their training over the next six weeks. Replace the fartlek workout with repeat intervals. Although there are myriad options regarding workouts, one plan is to alternate weekly speed sessions between 400-meter and 800-meter repeats. For either workout, be sure not to increase the distance of fast-paced running by more than a total of 800 meters per week. The speed of these repeats should be at their current race pace, performing an amount of recovery jogging equal to the repeated fast-paced segment.

Every third or fourth week, enter a 5K or 10K race to evaluate your training progress. Determine your race pace by checking the split times at each mile mark, or calculate your average mile pace from your overall finish time. You can then adjust the speed of future repeat intervals accordingly to allow for continued improvement.

Now is the time to tackle your target race. It is recommended that you taper the final week before the race by cutting your weekly mileage in half. Throw in a few 30-second bursts of speed to top off training during the last speed work session three to four days before the big event. During the race, focus on running an even but aggressive pace that you can maintain throughout the entire race. Turn on the afterburners the last 800 meters, and try to pass as many runners as possible while maintaining good running form.

Speed Work for the Experienced Runner

Although the base-building guidelines for all runners are the same, the experienced runner may find that she performs best at a level of 40–45 miles per week. Some advanced competitors even log weekly mileage at significantly higher levels. However, lingering leg fatigue and the increased risk of injury can outweigh the gain of running additional mileage run per week. Keep in mind that more is not always better, emphasizing running quality over quantity.

Many experienced runners can handle two advanced training workouts per week. Assuming a long run on Sunday, the advanced runner could do a fartlek workout on either Tuesdays or Wednesdays followed by a hill repeat workout on either Thursdays or Fridays the first four weeks of this phase of training. Listening to your body is the best way to determine which days your legs feel most rested and recovered for these advanced workouts. (Please refer to the guidelines provided earlier in this chapter on fartlek and hill repeats.)

For the first week, the fartlek workout would encompass 6 minutes of cumulative fast-paced efforts, adding 4 minutes per session for each of the next three weeks. Similarly, the hill repeats would begin with 6 charges up a

150–200 meter incline and adding 2 repeats per session for each of the next three weeks.

After completing four weeks of fartlek runs and hill repeats, you can begin more formal speed training (interval sessions) and continue these over the next eight to ten weeks. Again, assuming that your long run is Sunday, interval sessions could be performed either on Tuesdays or Wednesdays depending on what day your legs feel most rested. Your present 5K race pace determines how quickly you run these fast segments.

For the sake of this discussion, let's say that your present race pace is 8:00 per mile. In the first week of interval training, aim to run the 400-meter repeats at 7:40 pace per mile (1:55 per lap) followed by a 200-meter recovery jog. Repeat this sequence three more times, striving to run a consistent pace for each interval. The next week, run 800 meters at 7:50 pace per mile (3:55 for 2 laps) with a 400-meter recovery jog. Repeat this process two more times.

As your speed improves over the course of your race season, target the 400-meter repeat times to be approximately 20–25 seconds faster than your current 5K race pace. You should run the 800-meter repeats about 10–15 seconds faster than your 5K race pace. By the end of this phase of training, top out weekly interval sessions with workouts of 10–12 400-meter repeats and 5–6 800-meter repeats. Remember that with any speed workout or race, it is very important to include at least a 1–1½ mile warm-up and a 1-mile cool-down jog followed by 10–15 minutes of stretching.

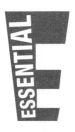

The experienced runner can also vary the interval workouts over the course of the next several weeks, beginning with longer repeat intervals during the earlier part of training (1,600 and 1,200 meters) and shortening the fast-paced segments as the target race grows closer. For variety, also include pyramids and ladder sessions among the possibilities in an interval session.

Along with interval sessions, the experienced runner might also want to include tempo workouts during this period of training. Tempo runs provide an opportunity to practice running at a fast pace for longer periods of time. These could be scheduled two to three days following the interval workout session or occasionally nested within a 10–12 mile run. The first week, aim to sustain a swift pace for 6 continuous minutes within the middle part of the workout, adding an additional 4 minutes for each subsequent week. Run the pace of the tempo segment approximately 10–15 seconds per mile slower than present 10K race pace.

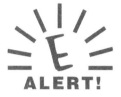
ALERT!

Reduce the strain on your knees (thus minimizing your risk of injury) when running on a track by changing your running direction midway through your speed workout. *Important:* Change directions only if no other runners or walkers are using the track. If you are running the workout with a group, make sure that the other runners also agree to do so.

Every third or fourth week, you can substitute a 5K or 10K practice race for a tempo workout or long run to evaluate training progress.

From these practice events, determine your current race pace (per mile) and adjust the speed of future repeat interval sessions accordingly to allow for continued improvement.

After the completion of the interval phase of training, you are now ready to race at your optimal level. Through the experience gained over the course of months and years of racing, advanced competitors better understand the maximum level they can push and maintain their race pace. Unlike the beginner and novice who often measure improvement in minutes, the experienced runner may only be able to improve by a few seconds from race to race.

Chapter 12

Completing a 10K and Half-Marathon

If you've come off some 5K races enjoying the experiences and eager for the next challenge, the 10K, or perhaps the half-marathon, is what you should set your sights on. The 10K doubles the 5K to 6.2 miles, and just as the 5K holds sufficient challenge for every level of runner, so the 10K is also a runner-friendly distance. If you're serious about your running and taking the advice of this book, you most certainly can bring your racing distance safely up from the 5K to the 10K and from there to the half-marathon (13.1 miles), while continuing to enjoy (almost) every minute of your races.

Mileage Buildup for the 10K

Once you've run a few 5Ks and have built a consistent running base, your objective may be to run a faster 5K race the next time out. If so, consider including in your training some of the advanced running workouts from Chapter 11 to help get you there. If you've yet to train for the 10K, however, your focus should be on handling the distance while running at a pace you can realistically maintain. Doing this successfully incorporates three elementals of being a runner: stamina, strength, and regulating of pace. Mastering these brings increased ability to all your runs and races.

In thinking about how to safely build your mileage to race the 10K, consult the Mileage Buildup Schedules in Chapter 5. There are two schedules—one for beginner and novice runners and one for advanced runners. Take a look at them to determine where you fit in based on your present running routine and your racing goals. Although both are designed to build you safely to running 10 miles, the beginner need not run more than 5 miles in training to be able to comfortably run a 10K race. On the other hand, experienced runners who have competitive aspirations for the 10K or who plan to run a longer event later in the race season may wish to build to the 10-mile level.

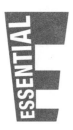

Tapering consists of a gradual decrease in running. For runners who race, this means cutting back on mileage in the week before a race. What's the advantage of this? It's so that on race day your legs are rested and you can do your best.

When you follow a training schedule specific to the goal of a race, as you should when training for a significant distance like the half-marathon or marathon, you will incorporate tapering time into your schedule. For shorter distances like the 5K or even the 10K, how much to taper depends on your goals, fitness level, and current weekly mileage.

Things to Consider When Increasing Your Distance

Remember that for the 10K you want to be able to handle the distance. You need leg strength, for sure, but you also need stamina and, if it's your goal, speed. Simply coming off of a 5K race in which you finished strong and felt good does not necessarily qualify you for doubling that distance— at least not competitively.

To set yourself up for equally enjoyable 10Ks, keep in mind this advice:

- **Form.** As you push yourself, don't get sloppy. It's better to put in fewer miles with proper form than to overexert yourself while running in such a way that could lead to injury. Pay particular attention to staying relaxed in your upper body.

- **Pace and time.** The 10K is a longer race and needs a different strategy from the 5K. You need reserves to push for a strong finish after running 6.2 miles, which is quite different from running 3.1 miles. One way to gauge the effectiveness of your training program for meeting your race goal(s) is to set up some mock 10Ks. Go the distance at approximately the same time of day in similar weather conditions, taking note of when you feel the strongest, when you feel like you're starting to lag, when you get your second wind, and so on. Be sure to wear your watch on all your runs so you can become better aware of pace and determine what pace is realistic for you.

- **Energy.** Energy comes from what you eat and drink, so be sure to be smart about both. (Review the advice in Chapter 9 so you are prepared for running in any weather.)

- **Safety.** When going out on longer runs, consider in advance the time of day you're running and what the environment is like. Wear reflective gear if there will be little light; carry a cell phone; be wary of road or trail conditions; and be mindful of staying hydrated.

- **Self-talk.** If running a longer distance seems intimidating, you may find yourself nagged by unreasonable fears. Change your self-talk so that you approach your runs with positive energy and enthusiasm. If your running program is realistic and your goals are within reason, you should be able to increase your mileage fairly easily.

- **Cool down.** Run the last half-mile or so of your long run slowly to help your body ease back into your regular routine.
- **Stretch.** As discussed throughout, a thorough stretch after a run is imperative, and especially so after a long run. Stretching helps your muscles recuperate and minimizes soreness later.

Running the 10K

When the big day finally arrives, you want to be ready for it. Prepare the way you would for any event, being sure to bring the supplies you need with you to the race, giving yourself plenty of time to register and warm up when you get there, using the facilities if necessary (and there are sometimes long lines for these!), and finding your place among the runners.

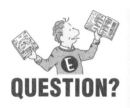

QUESTION?

How soon after my 10K can I run a 5K?
Depending on your mileage base, experience level, and how quickly you recover coming off the 10K, you could decide to compete in a 5K over the course of the weekends that follow. Running clubs sometimes hold seasonal race series in which they stage 5K races every week over the course of six to eight weeks. These are a good motivation for enjoying the experience of racing in an atmosphere of camaraderie.

Think about how competitive you want to be. If the race is your first 10K, you probably won't have winning as your goal. Decide on a time that you think is currently achievable for you in the race, and line up with the runners in that bracket. Posted behind the starting line at many races are signs indicating a continuum of anticipated paces that serve as a guide for runners to position themselves appropriately. It is important to place yourself based on a pace you can realistically maintain throughout the event—that is, where you won't slow others down or need to weave around those who might slow you down.

Once the race begins, settle into a pace based on your training runs for this distance. It's easy to excitedly start out too fast, especially if you feel fit and ready to tackle this new length. Rein yourself in a bit, thinking about how good you'll feel in the last few miles to have energy to draw upon in order to achieve your goal.

After the 10K

Your post-race routine should be fairly standardized by now: Spend a few minutes jogging easily or walking, drinking water, then stretching. Have a bagel, banana, or other nutritious snack. When you get home, shower, change, and you're ready for whatever your day or evening may bring!

In regard to your next race, the general formula is that for every mile raced, you should allow the same number of days before your next race. For example, if you run a 10K, then allow at least six to seven days before your next race. You'll probably feel better racing a 5K next; entering another 10K may be overdoing it. On the other hand, if you race a 5K the first weekend, doing a 10K the next could be a progressive step in your training. The success of either scenario depends on you as an individual and where you are in your training.

Training For and Running the Half-Marathon

The desire to race a half-marathon (13.1 miles) is a natural progression for many runners who have completed a mileage buildup program and wish to meet a new goal. Although it doesn't require the same degree of commitment as training for a marathon, the half-marathon is still a worthy challenge that many runners around the world seek. It's also a practical way to gauge your endurance if you're coming off racing the 10K and want to build up to a marathon.

Mileage Buildup for the Half-Marathon

Begin your half-marathon training by finding the training week or level from one of the two mileage buildup schedules in Chapter 5 that more closely matches your present training routine. From that point, proceed until you complete the remaining mileage specified on whichever schedule you use.

Next, continue your training by following your choice of the two schedules featured below. Determine the maximum distance of your longest training run (and thus your choice of charts) based on your competitive aspirations along with how much you enjoy doing long runs. You should complete the longest training run (16 miles) no more than three weeks before the half-marathon. Run at least 12 miles in practice to be minimally prepared for the 13.1-mile race.

Table 12-1

Novice Half-Marathon Training Schedule

Week #	Sun.	Mon.	Tue.	Wed.	Thur.	Fri.	Sat.	Total
1	11	Rest	5	7	5	Rest	5	33
2	12	Rest	5	7	5	Rest	5	34
3	8	Rest	6	Rest	4	Rest	2 Optional	18–20 Taper Week
4	13.1 (race day)	Rest	4	5	4	Rest	5	31

Advanced Half-Marathon Training Schedule

Week #	Sun.	Mon.	Tue.	Wed.	Thur.	Fri.	Sat.	Total
1	11	Rest	6	8	5	Rest	5	35
2	12	Rest	6	8	5	Rest	5	36
3	8	Rest	4	6	4	Rest	4	26 Easy Week
4	14	Rest	6	8	6	Rest	5	39
5	16	Rest	6	8	6	Rest	5	41
6	13	Rest	5	7	5	Rest	5	35
7	10	Rest	4	Rest	4	Rest	2 Optional	18–20 Taper Week
8	13.1 (race day)	Rest	4	6	4	Rest	4	31

Numbers refer to miles of running

The Long Run

While the long run is discussed in great detail in the marathon training chapters of this book (Chapters 17 and 18), the key points regarding this important workout are highlighted here. Similar to marathon training, the long run is the most important component of one's half-marathon training for teaching the body to both mentally and physically tackle the challenge of completing a race of 13.1 miles or longer. For the purpose of this discussion, the distance of a long run is considered to be 10 miles (or longer) or a run that lasts more than 90 minutes.

The long run also provides an excellent opportunity to experiment with a variety of concerns, such as shoes, nutrition, and pacing. Above all, long-distance training schedules must be designed so that runners are rested prior to undertaking their long runs. Runners who complete at least two long runs of 10 miles prior to a half-marathon are better prepared to face the challenge ahead of them.

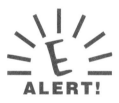
ALERT!

Don't split your long run! If your training schedule calls for a long run of 10 miles, you must run the distance at one time rather than splitting it into a 5-mile morning session and a 5-mile evening run.

The majority of runners who experience difficulty in completing their long training runs fail to prepare adequately for these critical workouts. The following guidelines enable you to prepare for and complete your long runs safely and successfully. Completing all your scheduled long runs, in turn, greatly enhances your chance of performing well on race day.

Pace and Time

Run at a conversational pace by starting out slowly to conserve glycogen. Your long-run pace should be approximately 1–1½ minutes slower than your present 10K race pace. You should be running so that your perceived exertion level seems easy and relaxed. Put another way, if you wished to carry on a lengthy conversation with another runner, you could easily do so without gasping for air.

There are two major reasons you need to run at a relaxed pace during the long run. Most important, you are conserving glycogen and glucose (your energy sources, converted from digested food stored in your working muscles and blood supply, respectively). Running at an easy pace also reduces the possibility of incurring an injury. This is particularly important since you are probably building your mileage to a level as yet unachieved. This in itself puts stress and strain on your muscles, joints, tendons, and ligaments.

As you focus on your pace, also consider running for cumulative time, approximating the distance you travel. For example, if your easy-run pace is 9 minutes per mile, run for 90 or so minutes for your 10-miler rather than finding a course that is exactly that distance. Doing so enables you to have more flexibility and spontaneity in regard to the route you choose to run. Schedule some long runs at the same time of day the actual race will be held to familiarize yourself with running during that time frame, and also to develop a pre-race routine that feels comfortable to you.

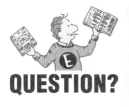

QUESTION?

Should I do long runs with others?
For your long runs, either run with friends or find a group running at your pace. Running with a group makes the long run more pleasurable and easier to accomplish than running alone.

Running Form and Upper Body Considerations

Although there is no need to alter your running stride, you need to focus on keeping your upper body relaxed and loose. Remember, tension is the adversary of all long-distance runners. Tension in the arms, shoulders, and especially the back drains energy and makes running more difficult. It creates stress that detracts from the main focus—running. Shake out your arms and shoulders regularly to combat tension.

Carry your arms close to your waist or hips to conserve energy. Also avoid unnecessary arm swing, particularly laterally across the body. Remember, this is wasted motion and energy expenditure, and it also puts extra strain on your hips.

Hydration

Water and sports drinks are your lifeline in completing these long runs. It is very important that you drink fluids every 25–30 minutes while you are running, regardless of weather conditions. For runs that are more than an hour long, you also need to drink sports drinks such as Gatorade or Powerade to fuel those working muscles, keeping them functioning optimally.

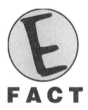

FACT

The half-marathon is an ideal race to use as a marathon tune-up. It provides an opportunity to experiment with a variety of factors, such as pre-race routine, nutrition, and pacing. Additionally, you can, to some extent, extrapolate your marathon finish time from the half-marathon distance. However, marathon predictor charts have less reliability if you haven't completed at least two runs of over 20 miles each.

Don't rely on your thirst mechanism to send a signal to your brain saying "I'm thirsty!" If you wait until that point, you will not be able to consume enough fluids to catch up with your hydration needs. Doing so puts you at greater risk of heat illness. (Check out Chapter 9 for more information on running in the heat.) In short, dehydration is one of your biggest enemies. Many beginners fail to grasp this and ignore opportunities to take in fluids. Don't pass these up. Drink!

Psychological Issues

Realize that long runs are sometimes difficult to complete and that you may experience some bad patches in the later miles. Persevering through these stretches helps you to develop mental toughness, a skill that is essential during a half-marathon or a full marathon. Use imagery, mental rehearsal or visualization, and self-talk to develop mental toughness. For example, to make the run seem more doable, try to mentally break the course into sections. That is, mentally run from one landmark to the next instead of thinking of completing the entire 10-mile training course. When you reach the first landmark, then mentally think of running to the next, and so forth.

If this seems like a real hurdle to you, review the sections in Chapter 8 on yoga and meditation. These are practices proven to help athletes stay focused and run better, with improved breathing techniques and mental acuity.

A cardinal rule of long-distance racing is: Don't try anything new or leave anything to chance on race day. Use all training runs as opportunities for experimentation. For a variety of issues on which you should consider experimenting long before race weekend arrives, see the final section of this chapter, "Runners, Take Your Mark, Set, Race!"

Finally, after the run is over, continue to drink fluids (water, sports drinks, and juice are all good choices). Also, eat some more; you've earned it! As soon as possible (ideally within 15 minutes of the end of the run), have something to eat to replace depleted glycogen stores. Research has shown that to avoid muscle fatigue the next day, carbohydrates should be eaten as soon as possible following long-duration exercise.

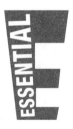

You might want to engage in some other activities after completing your long run and half-marathon. Do some light cycling or walking later in the day to loosen up your legs. Also consider using therapeutic techniques such as dipping your legs in cool water immediately after the run or getting a leg massage over the next couple of days to reduce muscle soreness and fatigue.

Runners, Take Your Marks, Set, Race!

For the sake of discussion, assume that your half-marathon race is scheduled for Sunday at 8:00 A.M. By experimenting with concerns during your long training runs, you greatly increase the chance that your half-marathon experience will be a successful one.

First, you need to get lots of rest Saturday night. Aim for at least eight hours of sleep. What you don't want to do is tire out your legs, so make either Friday or Saturday a complete rest day for the legs. If you must train, do something light (not a run). If you train on Saturday, make it a very light workout on the legs. If your friends want to go dancing, ask them to reschedule for the following week.

What to Eat and Drink

What you drink and eat can make a big difference in your performance on race day. First, drink lots of water. You have to fight the possibility of dehydration, so drink water all day Saturday. (It is possible to drink too much water, so be careful.) Additionally, you can eat a lot, but make sure you eat smart. Eat meals high in carbohydrates for lunch and dinner Saturday, but don't eat the wrong foods. Select the right pre-race meal for you, such as pasta with marinara sauce as opposed to Alfredo sauce. Avoid foods high in salt, excessive protein, and fat all day Saturday. Also, this may surprise you, but go light on salads and vegetables; these can cause a host of digestive problems.

On Sunday morning, drink about sixteen ounces of water prior to your race. Additionally, eat a light snack. Figure out what you must eat and how early to do so to avoid digestive problems.

While running, you want to drink lots of fluids. Be sure to stop for water frequently throughout the run. For runs and races longer than 90 minutes, you should strive to drink sports beverages every 2–3 miles or every 25–30 minutes. Drinking on the run requires careful planning of the route (make sure there is water available frequently, along with places to stash sports drinks). Most races have frequent water stops, and almost all (with the exception of some 5Ks) provide sports drinks.

You may also want to consider using gel carbohydrate replacement products during the run. Be sure to chase them down with water to avoid stomach cramps and to enhance the absorption of these products. (Please dispose of gel and energy wrappers properly by throwing them away in trash receptacles or placing them in your fanny pack. There's nothing worse than a disrespectful runner.)

Shoes, Apparel, and Accessories

You should remember that, especially for a long run, good equipment is essential. To get through the race comfortably, pay particular attention to your shoes, apparel, and accessories.

For your footwear, make sure that your shoes have low mileage to maximize absorption of shock. Do not wear new shoes or shoes that are not sufficiently broken in for a long run or race. On the other hand, make sure the shoes you wear aren't broken down.

In addition to shoes, comfortable and functional clothing is one of the most important ingredients for runs of all distances, particularly for long runs and races. Wear Coolmax or synthetic-blend socks, singlets, shorts, and leggings that wick away moisture and won't cause chafing. Again, don't wear anything for the first time at the race. Wear socks and other apparel that you have worn at least once during training and that have been washed. Also, remember to use Skin-Lube or Vaseline (on feet, under arms, between thighs, nipples, etc.) to eliminate or reduce chafing and/or blisters.

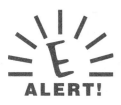
ALERT!

When dressing for a run, remember that excess clothing causes overheating of the body. Once you begin running, it will feel as if the outside temperature has risen by 10 degrees. Also remember that hats trap body heat, making them perfect for a cold weather race but a bad idea for a race with hot and humid conditions.

When the Race Is Over

You mean you have to do something after the run is over? Yes! Sometimes injuries occur as a result of not giving your fatigued muscles the cool-down they need and deserve. Follow these three simple guidelines after every long-distance run, and you'll feel better.

Drink and Eat

You've sweated the miles, you've burned off the calories, you've earned it. There will probably be food available from the race organizers when you reach the finish line. After stretching, enjoy a bagel, a banana, or a cup of soup—or all three. When you get home, you may be hungry again. Although this isn't an invitation to pig-out and throw all dietary caution to the wind, the maxims "I eat, therefore I run" and "Eat, drink, and be merry" each apply in moderation.

Cool Down

Cool down by running the last half-mile slowly. Or once you've crossed the finish line, walk for awhile or jog another half-mile to slow your body down. It may sound crazy, but your body will in fact feel better for it.

Stretch

After you've walked a little and had something to drink, stretch thoroughly while your muscles are still warm. This can't be stated strongly enough, since your muscles will probably be tight from the long distance that you've covered. Don't wait until you've cooled off or you're more likely to hurt yourself. Also, stretching warm muscles helps make them less stiff and painful later on in the day.

Chapter 13

Injury Prevention

The majority of running injuries occur from training errors. To avoid injury, your increase in mileage and speed should be gradual. It is important to intersperse hard days and easy days as well as hard and easy weeks. You should increase mileage approximately 10 percent per week, and every fourth week you should back off slightly.

Avoiding Injury: The Basics

Most runners should devote at least one or two days a week to rest or non-running activities. That gives your body a chance to recover and strengthen itself. It is also helpful to maintain a running diary, which should contain your mileage, course, and brief notes on how you felt during each run. Such a record can help trace the origin of any number of training errors.

Not only do your mileage, frequency of running, the course you run, and the times you post matter, there are other factors that contribute to how you feel and how your training progresses. You will find that taking note of physical infirmities like a scratchy throat, headache, or bloated feeling can help you pinpoint when you started coming down with something more serious.

Treating Inflammation

Inflammation (characterized by pain, swelling, redness, and warmth) is often a byproduct of injury. If inflammation occurs in an injury site, treat the area with ice (see icing guidelines below). Above all, do not treat the area with heat of any kind, wet or dry, for several days.

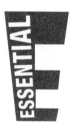

The medications you take can affect your running, as can time changes when you travel, dietary changes, and increased stress on the job or at home. Your running diary may become so much more to you than a simple record, leaving you amazed when you look back after a year has gone by.

Consider taking several days off from running as well as from any other sports that cause stress to the injured area. Try taking some anti-inflammatory medication (such as ibuprofen, naproxen sodium, or acet-aminophen) for the injury, being careful to follow dosing instructions to avoid internal problems.

Icing can also be helpful. Apply ice to the area for 20 minutes and repeat once an hour for three times on the first few evenings after an injury. Heat is a relaxing therapeutic measure after significantly reducing or eliminating inflammation of the injury site. Applying a hot water bottle wrapped in a towel or a special sports pad that can be microwaved warm or soaking in a hot tub can bring relief to minor injuries on the mend. But be sure to not overdo it, though, since heat can also result in swelling.

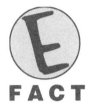

FACT

To properly ice an injury, use an ice cup. Fill a small paper cup with water and then place it in the freezer. When completely frozen, the top of the paper cup can be peeled away to expose the ice. As the ice applied to the injury melts, continue to push the ice through the opening. Massage the injured area with the ice cup for approximately 10 minutes or until the area is numb. Ice the area again 2–3 hours later (or as often as possible).

If all these remedies fail, consider visiting a physician familiar with sports injuries and experience treating runners to obtain an assessment of the injury and treatment advice. (Details on how to find a sports physician are at the end of this chapter.) The most important information a physician can provide is whether you: can continue to run without modification of your training schedule; can continue to run with a reduced workload; must rest the injury site (that is, no running); and/or should add cross-training activities both to maintain cardiovascular fitness and to strengthen the injury site.

The Impact (Literally!) of Athletic Shoes

As discussed in Chapter 3, running shoes should be replaced regularly. The shock-absorbing capability of the midsole diminishes gradually and becomes inadequate after 350–500 miles. The number of miles depends on such factors as your weight, the training terrain, and environmental conditions. Even if the upper part of the shoe does not show much wear, the shock absorption may already be gone. If you are running approximately 20 miles per week, you should be replacing your shoes between four and six months, depending upon your shock absorption needs. Use your runner's diary to note the condition of your running shoes. If you decide to change brands for any reason, you can track your comments as well as compare shoe performance.

Even if you are a careful runner, stretching consistently and not overextending yourself in your runs, you can incur injury from running in poorly designed shoes. By recognizing potential problems associated with faulty shoe design, you become a more discerning shoe buyer and ensure that the shoes you are wearing meet your biomechanical needs.

Shoes and Achilles Tendonitis

Shoes with inflexible soles cause the calf muscles to work harder and can contribute to the development of *Achilles tendonitis,* in which the Achilles tendon becomes inflamed. The mechanical reason for this is best explained by looking at the foot as a fulcrum and lever system. Shoes with inflexible soles make the lever arm (the foot) function over a longer distance and make the tip of the shoe the location of the fulcrum (the pivot point). Ideally, the shoe should flex at the point where the toes join the foot (which also happens to be the widest part of the shoe), offering more support. The shoes should also have a slight heel lift, which most running shoes do.

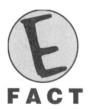

FACT

Don't even dream of running a marathon in a new pair of shoes. Your shoes should have at least 70 miles logged on them (including one long training run of 20 miles or longer) to be broken in well enough to run a marathon.

Shoes that have too much heel cushioning, including some air-cushioned models, can also contribute to Achilles tendonitis. After the heel strikes the ground, it continues moving as the shoe's cushioning continues to absorb shock. This continued motion can stretch a susceptible Achilles tendon excessively.

Shoes and Plantar Fasciitis

Running shoes too flexible in the midsole or that flex before the point at which the toes join the foot can both stretch the *plantar fascia* (the bowstring-like tissue on the sole of your foot) and contribute to excessive pronation in the foot. The resulting lack of stability occurs not just in the shoe's transverse plane (where the shoe actually flexes), but also in its longitudinal plane, thereby reducing the effectiveness of the shoe in controlling pronation.

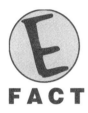

FACT

Make sure you carefully lace your shoes before running. Too tight a shoe can make the top of your foot sore or squeeze your *metatarsals* too tightly. This in turn can result in feelings of numbness and/or tingling in your feet, particularly on long training runs. Too loose a shoe can make your foot less stable, resulting in excessive pronation and increasing the possibility of blisters.

Tips for Buying and Wearing Shoes

A shoe's midsole degrades from use. Given the lifespan of a running shoe (350–500 miles, maximum), if you are running about 20 miles a week, you should consider changing shoes at weeks 20–25. Although the shoes are no longer good for running, they can still serve as casual wear for walking.

When assessing the condition of your running shoes, realize that even a new-looking shoe might lack adequate shock absorption. Use the 350–500 mile guideline instead of trying to guess how worn your shoes should look.

When buying your running shoes, make sure there is about a thumb's width of space between your big toe and the material at the very front of the shoe (called the toe box). This helps prevent runner's (black) toe and/or losing your toenails. It's also important that the shape and depth of the toe box is spacious enough to prevent the toes from rubbing on the top and sides of the shoe.

If you have had no problems while running in a shoe, you should probably buy another pair of the same make and model. Should that model be discontinued by the manufacturer (a very common occurrence), see whether it's available through a running specialty store or look at ads in the back of a magazine like *Runner's World*.

Guide to Shoes and Foot-Related Problems

The following lists appropriate shoe designs for certain foot conditions:

- **Low arch:** This condition needs much support, so choose a stable shoe with good rear foot control.
- **High arch:** This problem needs more shock absorption, meaning you will do better with a narrower heel.
- **Normal foot:** This is ideal, so you'll do well with a shoe that combines control and shock absorption.
- **Post-stress fracture:** A fracture requires you to change your shoes frequently (350–500 miles) and to buy shoes with adequate shock absorption.
- **Achilles tendonitis:** Tendonitis necessitates avoiding air soles, excessively spongy heels, and stiff soles as well as using a heel lift.

Stretching to Prevent Injuries

As discussed at length in Chapter 7, stretching cannot be emphasized enough as an injury-preventive routine. Runners frequently develop tightness in the posterior muscle groups, which include the hamstrings and calf muscles. The quadriceps and anterior shin muscles can become relatively weak due to muscular imbalance. The abdominal muscles also tend to be weak on runners who do not exercise them.

The Magic Six, Plus Two

George Sheehan recommends a revised set of "Magic Six" stretches in his columns and in his book *Running to Win* (Rodale Press, 1991). Following is a slightly modified version of Dr. Sheehan's Magic Six, Plus Two.

1. The *wall pushup* is a calf stretch that stretches one leg at a time. Stand with your rear foot approximately 2–3 feet from the wall. Your rear leg should be straight, your front leg bent, and your hands touching the wall. Point feet straight ahead, heels on the ground. Hold for 30 seconds; switch legs.

2. Next is the *hamstring stretch.* Straighten one leg, placing it with knee locked on a foot stool. Bend your body and bring your head toward the leg. Hold this position for 30 seconds and switch sides.

3. In addition to the hamstring stretch, you can also try the *knee clasp* by lying on a firm surface (a carpeted floor or grass is best). Bring both knees to your chest and hold for 30 seconds. This stretches the hamstrings and lower back.

4. Another excellent stretch is the *chest pushup.* Lie face down on the floor with your abdomen pressed flat against the floor. Place your hands flat on the floor, beneath your shoulders. Push your chest up with your arms, and hold for 30 seconds.

5. To do the *backward stretch,* you simply place the palms of your hands against the small of your back while standing straight. Tighten your buttocks, and bend backward. Hold for 30 seconds.

6. The *shin splinter* is a stretch to strengthen the shins. Sit on a table with your legs dangling over the side. Place a 3–5 pound weight on your toes. Flex your foot at the ankle (bending it up). Hold for 6 seconds; repeat five times.

7. To strengthen the *quadriceps*, do straight-leg lifts. Lying on the floor, flex one knee at approximately a right angle. Lift the other leg rapidly between 30°–60°. Lower and repeat ten times. Switch legs, repeat five times, and work up to ten sets of ten repetitions.

8. Finally, the *bent leg sit-up* strengthens the abdominals. Dr. Sheehan recommends the sit-up be a gradual one rather than a rapid thrust forward. It should feel as if you are moving forward one vertebra at a time. Lie on

the floor with your knees bent. Sit up thirty degrees from the floor. Lie back, and then repeat twenty times.

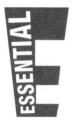

Since hardly any runner wants to perform eight stretches (even if disguised as six plus two!), the four exercises you should do for optimal health and injury prevention are the wall pushup, hamstring stretch, knee clasp, and bent leg sit-up. Do straight-leg lifts if you have runner's knee.

Avoid Overstretching

Even as many runners neglect stretching, some in fact overstretch, perhaps in response to injury. This is not always a good thing.

If you are currently injured, now is not a good time to start stretching since this can further tear a muscle or tendon fiber. If your Achilles tendon is sore, don't start on a high-intensity stretching program to try to improve it. A sign that stretching is contraindicated is an increase in pain as a result. Let your muscle heal a bit before trying to stretch it.

Instead, use a heel lift, avoid hills, decrease your stride, and discard shoes that use a gas in the heel for shock absorption. Decrease the intensity and duration of your training runs. Once you are feeling better, probably in about three to six weeks, you can begin a light and easy stretching regimen. The same rationale holds for other injured body parts.

The Gait Biomechanics of Foot and Leg Problems

To understand lower leg problems runners encounter, you should be aware of how biomechanical abnormalities in the lower body are related to specific foot and leg problems. The following is a review of the gait cycle, which leads to a more complex discussion of foot and lower leg biomechanics.

Many specific foot problems are caused by biomechanical faults within the foot or lower leg. In order to understand the cause of these problems, it helps to have a working knowledge of the normal anatomy, function, and biomechanics of the lower leg. By visualizing the events of the normal gait cycle during walking or running and breaking these down into phases and subphases, each action of the foot and leg can be evaluated at a specific sequential time period.

Anatomy of the Gait

Before understanding the specifics of gait, take a brief look at the bones involved. The key bone structures are the *talus* and *calcaneus* (located at the ankle and comprising the subtalar joint) and the *navicular* and *cuboid* (located just forward of these bones). The talus and navicular along with the calcaneus and cuboid make up what is known as the *midtarsal* joint. The leg bones of significance consist of the *femur* (the thigh bone) and the *tibia* (the larger of the two lower leg bones). The *fibular* is the smaller leg bone. In front of the tibia is the *patella,* or kneecap.

Phases of Gait

The gait cycle of each leg is divided into the *stance phase* and the *swing phase.* The stance phase is the period during which the foot is in contact with the ground; the swing phase is the period in which the foot is off the ground and swinging forward.

In walking, the stance phase comprises approximately 60 percent of the gait cycle and the swing phase about 40 percent. The proportion of swing to stance phase changes as the speed of walking or running increases. As the speed is increased, the percentage of time spent in the stance phase decreases. Increased time is then spent in the swing phase, with a corresponding increase in the importance of swing phase muscles.

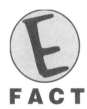

FACT

It is important to note that, in running, a third subphase is present, called the *float phase.* During the float phase, neither foot is on the ground.

Stance and Swing Phases of Gait

The stance phase comprises 40 percent of the gait cycle in running, compared with 60 percent of the gait cycle in walking. The time period during which the foot is in contact with the ground and the resulting forces differ dramatically between running and walking. A walker moving at a comfortable speed of 120 steps per minute has a total gait cycle time of 1 second. A runner moving at 12 miles per hour has a cycle time of 0.6 second, even though the stance phase decreases from .62 second to 0.2 seconds.

The stance phase can be further subdivided into three subphases. The first component of the stance phase is called *heel contact*. This subphase begins when the heel makes contact with the ground and is completed when the remainder of the foot touches the ground. During this portion of the stance phase, the foot is pronating at the *subtalar joint*. The leg is internally rotating while the foot is absorbing shock and functioning as a mobile adaptor to the ground surface.

The next portion of the stance phase is called *midstance*. Midstance subphase begins when the entire foot contacts the ground. The body weight passes over the foot as the tibia and the rest of the body move forward. The opposite leg is off the ground and the foot bears the body weight alone. During this subphase, the leg is externally rotating and the foot is supinating at the subtalar joint. The foot changes from being a mobile adaptor to becoming a rigid lever in order to propel the body forward during the final component of the stance phase, known as *propulsion*.

Propulsion begins after the heel is off the ground (heel off) and ends when the toe is off the ground (toe off). This subphase constitutes the final 35 percent of stance phase. The body is propelled forward during this subphase, while weight is shifted to the opposite foot as it makes ground contact. The subtalar joint must be in a supinated position in order for this subphase to be normal and efficient. If abnormal pronation is occurring, the midstance subphase and this propulsion subphase are probably prolonged, with the result that weight transfer through the forefoot is not normal.

The swing phase begins immediately after toe off. The first component of the swing phase is the *forward swing*, which occurs as the foot is being carried forward. The knee is flexed, and the foot is flexed at this time. The next segment of the swing phase is called *foot descent,* in which the foot is positioned for weight bearing and the muscles stabilize the body to absorb the shock of heel contact. At heel contact the swing phase ends, and a new gait cycle begins.

In normal walking, the foot initially contacts the ground at the heel. The major determinant of where maximum heel wear occurs is based on the initial point of contact. The direction that your toes point has the greatest influence on this. If the toes point outward from the center of your body, your shoe will almost always strike the ground initially on the outer (lateral) portion of the heel. Medial heel wear likely indicates a gait in which the toes point in and usually occurs when there is rotational abnormality in the limb above.

In the gait of much faster speeds, such as sprinting, there may be no initial heel contact. An individual might make contact at midfoot and then rock backwards onto the heel or not touch the heel down at all.

From Gait to Feet to Legs

Now that you understand the basic phases of gait, you can learn to recognize the motions of the legs and feet and the interrelationship of these structures. The period of double support, during which both feet are on the ground, occurs twice during the stance phase, during the initial portion and in the final 20 percent.

The terminal double support phase has implications for the final portion of stance phase, which is the propulsion subphase. The propulsion subphase can be divided into active and passive periods. The active portion occurs after heel off yet before the opposite foot touches down and terminal double support begins. The passive portion of terminal double support begins with the touchdown of the opposite foot and the ending of the work that the propelling calf muscle was doing. Some people call this subphase the pre-swing phase.

At heel contact, the pelvis is slightly in external rotation. Slightly after heel contact, as the foot is adapting to the ground, the pelvis rotates internally. Just before toe off, it rotates externally, where it remains during the swing phase.

Force Flow

Force flow through the foot can today be measured by a variety of means. The Electrodynogram, the first system available for doctor's office use, consisted of seven sensors applied to standard positions on the foot. Other technology exists today that accomplishes this and lets you observe forces beneath the foot that normally cannot be seen. Devices also measure the timing of the phases and subphases of gait, greatly increasing knowledge of what is occurring during the gait cycle. Normal pressure flow through the foot starts slightly lateral in the heel, flows forward between the first and second metatarsi, and exits through the big toe.

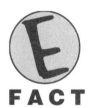

FACT

During running, if a runner swings his arms across his body, there is a compensatory increase in pelvic rotation. It is more efficient for the pelvis and better for the pelvic musculature if the runner moves his arms parallel to the motion in which he is running.

Selecting a Sports Physician

It is important to choose a doctor with experience in treating athletes. You cannot rely on finding such a doctor simply by referencing a telephone book. The best sources of information are other runners. Ask around; chances are high that several members of an area running club have needed treatment from a specialist sports doctor. A specialty running store is another source since the employees there are typically runners. Even if they're not, they should be able to put you in touch with individuals or groups that can help you. Why go to all this trouble? Because it is vital that you choose a medical specialist with both experience and a good reputation among runners.

Board Certification

Despite suggestions in the popular press that your sports physician be board-certified in sports medicine, there are no organizations that currently award such certification to any physician, including podiatric physicians.

Fellowship status can be achieved, however, through qualification and testing by the American College of Sports Medicine and the American Academy of Podiatric Sports Medicine.

A *Certificate of Added Qualifications in Sports Medicine* is granted physicians who meet multiple criteria and successfully pass a certifying examination given through a joint venture of the American Board of Family Practice, American Board of Podiatrics, American Board of Internal Medicine, and American Board of Emergency Medicine.

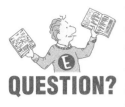

QUESTION?

Should the sports physician be a runner, too?
Whether the doctor is also a runner doesn't matter. Although a doctor-athlete can add to your understanding of the psychical and physical conditions that lead to injury, this is not a prerequisite for appropriate diagnosis and treatment. The recommendations of knowledgeable people are the most valuable resource for finding a capable sports medicine physician.

Other sports medicine organizations include the American Orthopedic Society of Sports Medicine and the American Medical Society of Sports Medicine. Organizations that can help you find a capable sports medicine practitioner are the American Running and Fitness Association, the American Academy of Podiatric Sports Medicine, and the American College of Sports Medicine.

Chapter 14

Injuries of the Foot and Ankle

It is beyond the scope of this book to discuss in detail the nature and treatment of most running injuries without knowing the symptoms. However, in order to give a practical overview of as many common injuries as possible, this chapter focuses alphabetically on injuries of the foot and ankle. Chapter 15 addresses injuries of the leg and other parts of the body directly affected by running.

General Injury Guidelines

Should you run with an injury? Perhaps, as long as you can run at a level of intensity below the threshold of pain without altering your normal running stride. When an injury occurs, reduce your mileage and intensity until you can resume running without pain. Do not take medication or ice an injury before testing whether or not you can run, since doing so would only mask the injury and possibly make it worse.

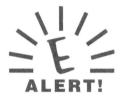
ALERT!

If something hurts, do not run; instead, choose a cross-training activity to maintain cardiovascular fitness. The following sports are generally safe for injured runners: walking, elliptical training, cycling, swimming, deep-water running, rowing, elliptical training, and Pilates. If you must stop running altogether for more than a week, ease back into your running slowly.

Recognize the difference between fatigue and pain due to an injury. Unfortunately, feel-good endorphins (the chemicals the body produces from aerobic exercise) mask pain. Listen to your body, and respect what it is telling you.

Some minor discomforts go away once muscles warm up. Be very cautious in this case, for you don't want to cause more serious damage to an injury site. Above all, if pain becomes more intense while running, do not continue. Instead, walk and begin treatment.

Achilles Tendonitis

Achilles tendonitis is the bane of many runners. The Achilles tendon is what connects the heel with the most powerful muscle group in the body, located in the back of your lower leg. It is the hard line you feel behind your ankle. The Achilles tendon joins three muscles—the two heads of the *gastrocnemius* and the *soleus*. The gastrocnemius heads arise from the posterior portion of the *femoral condyles*. The soleus arises from the posterior aspect of the tibia and fibula.

The gastrocnemius is a muscle that crosses three joints: the knee, the ankle, and the subtalar joint. The functioning of these joints and the influence of other muscles on these joints has a significant effect on the tension that occurs within the Achilles tendon. For example, tight hamstrings impact the functioning of the ankle joint and the subtalar joint and increase tension in the Achilles tendon. The soleus, on the other hand, does not cross the knee.

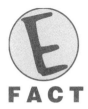

FACT

The Achilles tendon does not have a rich blood supply. It is not invested within a true tendon sheath; therefore, the blood supply to the proximal portion of the tendon comes from the branches of the muscles themselves.

What Causes Achilles Tendonitis

Chronic Achilles tendonitis arises from ignoring pain in your Achilles tendon and continuing to run. If your Achilles tendon is getting sore, you should immediately attend to it.

Sudden increases in training can contribute to Achilles tendonitis, particularly excessive hill running or a sudden addition of hills and speed work.

Two shoe construction flaws can also aggravate Achilles tendonitis. The first is a sole that is too stiff, especially at the ball of the foot. This means the "lever arm" of the foot is longer and the Achilles tendon is under increased tension, forcing the calf muscles to work harder to lift your heel off the ground.

The second shoe factor that can lead to a chronic Achilles tendon problem is excessive heel cushioning. Air-filled heels, which supposedly are nowadays more resistant to deformation and leaks, are not good for a sore Achilles tendon. The reason for this is quite simple. If you are wearing a shoe designed to give superior heel shock absorption, what frequently happens is that after heel contact, your heel continues to sink lower while your shoe is absorbing the shock. This further stretches the Achilles tendon at a moment when the leg and the rest of the body are moving forward over the foot. Change your shoes to one without this feature. Make sure to avoid training in racing flats if you have Achilles tendonitis.

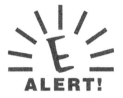

ALERT!

Another major contributor to Achilles tendonitis is excessive tightness of the posterior leg muscles—the calf muscles and the hamstrings. Do not perform gentle calf stretching, even though this may seem to be good for the area. The truth is that excessive stretching is not good for your Achilles tendon. In most cases, stretches put too much tension on an already tender Achilles tendon. A wall stretch is a good exception.

Treating Achilles Tendonitis

If you are suffering from Achilles tendonitis, the first thing to do is to cut back your training. If you are working out twice a day, change to once a day and take one or two days off per week. If you are working out every day, cut back to every other day and decrease your mileage. Training modification is essential to treatment of this potentially long-lasting problem.

You should also cut back on hill work and speed work. Applying ice after running may also help. Be sure to avoid excessive stretching. Accompany the first phase of healing with relative rest, which doesn't necessarily mean stopping running, but just cut back in training. If this does not help quickly, consider having a quarter-inch heel lift put into your shoe. Do not worry that you will become dependent on this; instead, concentrate on getting rid of the pain. Don't walk barefoot around your house and avoid excessively flat shoes, such as sneakers, tennis shoes, cross trainers, and so on.

Clinical treatment of Achilles tendonitis initially consists of the physical therapy modalities of electrical stimulation (HVGS, or high voltage galvanic stimulation) and ultrasound. Your sports physician should also carefully check your shoes. A heel lift can also be used and taping can control excessive pronation. These methods can be incorporated in a program of Achilles tendonitis rehabilitation therapy. Orthotics with a small heel lift are often helpful.

When the Achilles Tendon Ruptures

A ruptured or torn Achilles tendon is a very serious and potentially permanently debilitating injury that requires extreme care to repair and heal. If you suspect this has happened to you, read carefully and consult a trusted sports physician as soon as possible.

What actually causes the Achilles tendon to rupture is not entirely known, though it is associated with overworking unused or overused muscles. It is a common injury of weekend warriors who don't exercise consistently but overexercise on the weekend, though it can happen to seasoned athletes as well. The mechanism of injury is a force that increases the tension in the tendon beyond its tensile strength. A forceful stretch of the tendon or a contraction of the muscles can create this force. Most often, it is a combination of the two forces.

Occasionally, ruptures occur at the tendon-bone interface or within a 3–5 centimeter area above the tendon's insertion point. Since vascularity decreases with age, this frequently occurs in older athletes. A weakening of the Achilles tendon has been observed following intra-tendinous steroid injection. Therefore, injections of steroids are not recommended at this location. Diseases associated with an increased incidence of tendon rupture include gout, systemic lupus erythematosis, rheumatoid arthritis, and tuberculosis.

Diagnosing a Ruptured Achilles

Physical examination of the site of a recent rupture may reveal a noticeable gap. Swelling is observed. The most frequently described clinical test is called the Thompson test. As you lie on your stomach, your calf is squeezed. Your foot will plantar flex (raise the heel) if you do not have a completely torn Achilles tendon. The foot will not plantar flex when the Achilles tendon is completely torn. An MRI will accurately reveal the extent of the tear. Diagnostic ultrasound is also used to assist in the diagnosis of a torn Achilles tendon.

Treating a Ruptured Achilles Tendon

Complete tears of the Achilles tendon are usually treated with surgical repair followed by up to twelve weeks in a series of casts. Partial tears are sometimes treated with casting alone for up to twelve weeks and sometimes treated as complete tears, with surgery and casting. A heel lift is usually used for six months to one year following removal of the cast. Rehabilitation to regain flexibility and then to regain muscle strength is also instituted following removal of the cast.

Ankle Sprains

Ankle sprains are more common in athletes participating in sports with side-to-side movement than in those with straight-ahead motion. Court sports such as basketball, tennis, and racquetball all spawn their fair share of ankle sprains. Running on level ground does not often result in an ankle sprain, but cross-country running, trail running, stepping in a pothole, or missing the curb can all potentially lead to an ankle sprain. The most frequent ankle sprain is an inversion ankle sprain. This can injure the outer structures of the ankle.

The most common ankle injury resulting from an inversion is a partial tear of the *anterior talo-fibular ligament.* This ligament may also tear completely. The next most frequently injured ligament is the *calcaneo-fibular ligament.* The least injured is the *posterior talo-fibular ligament.* On occasion, the fibula itself may be fractured or the talar dome injured. The other structures on the lateral side of the ankle should always be carefully examined to make sure they are not injured.

The grading of ankle sprains is officially done on an inadequate three-point scale. Grade 1 is a mild stretch of ligament(s), Grade 3 is a complete tear of ligament(s), and Grade 2 is everything in between.

Treatment for Minor Sprains

It is impossible to guess how badly injured you are. If you have doubts or if your ankle swells very rapidly, you should head for an emergency room. Immediate treatment should consist of RICE: Rest, Ice, Compression (gentle), and Elevation. The ice should be applied for about 15 minutes at a time and then off for about the same. Avoid damaging your skin with the chemical bags you can place in your freezer. A bag of frozen corn or peas works just fine. If your ankle does not respond quickly to this treatment, it is probably best to visit your sports physician for an evaluation and treatment.

For Grade 2 sprains, an air cast is sometimes recommended to hold the ankle quiet as it heals and to prevent further tearing or strain. A removable walking cast, called a pneumatic walker, is used to provide stability and to allow you to bear weight without pain while keeping your ankle in a stable and secure position.

Starting to Exercise the Injury

The first exercise to try once your ankle starts to feel better is dorsiflexion-plantarflexion, or just plain moving the ankle up and down. After more improvement, moving in small circles, painting the alphabet with your toes and other exercises can be done. Later still, you can use a theraband or other elastic band to strengthen the muscles that help hold your ankle stable. Don't force your ankle to move in pain too soon, and avoid weight bearing or walking in pain early in the course of an ankle sprain. There is no reason to start testing your ankle until it has had time to heal. Slow and easy gains more than rushing into painful exercises. One way to see if you are ready to resume your full exercise regimen is to try to rapidly go downstairs without limping, pain, or any hitches in how you feel overall.

Anterior Ankle Pain

The tendons in front of your ankle can sometimes become irritated when the shoe tongue continues up around the front of the ankle and is compressed by the laces. This can also impinge upon the nerves in this area, resulting in an occasional numbness, but often pain. Of course, injuries to ligaments or bones can also cause pain in this area. Try skipping the top lace completely rather than lacing it looser. You can then lace your shoe securely without irritation. Odds are this should help a lot. If this simple solution doesn't work, get your ankle checked by a sports medicine practitioner.

Athlete's Foot

You don't have to be an athlete to have athlete's foot (*tinea pedis*). The condition got its name because it is spread in warm, moist places such as locker rooms. Athlete's foot is actually caused by a fungus or a type of mold, less often by a yeast. Fungus flourishes in dark, warm, moist environments. Shoes, being an occlusive covering of the foot, can be like a fungal heaven.

Clinical Appearance of Athlete's Foot

Athlete's foot can appear as cracked and peeling skin between the toes or on the bottom of the foot. It is often itchy but not always. Sometimes the flaking, scaling, or dry skin that you think is just a bit of excessive dryness is in reality evidence of athlete's foot. Small blisters may occur in conjunction with some fungal infections.

Between the toes the skin can become macerated or excessively soft and mushy. The fungus can go deeper into the skin through cracks or breaks, so that bacteria enters and causes a more troubling secondary bacterial infection.

Preventing Athlete's Foot

As with many things, the best cure is prevention. Since moisture is a risk factor, keeping your feet dry is important. Make sure you dry your feet carefully after showers. In the locker room, consider wearing shower sandals to limit exposure to any areas contaminated with fungus. Be careful to dry between your toes, and make sure your feet are dry before putting on your socks. You might sprinkle an antifungal foot powder in your shoes or on your feet.

Another important thing to remember is that cotton socks hold moisture against the foot rather than allowing it to readily evaporate. Make sure you wear socks made of noncotton material that wicks moisture away from the foot.

Treating Athlete's Foot

Mild fungal infections can be treated with over-the-counter medicine readily found in your pharmacy. Stubborn fungal infections require prescription-strength medicine. Make certain you follow directions for prevention to avoid a recurrence and to speed up elimination of the fungal infection. Keeping your feet dry is key to eliminating and preventing reinfection.

Heel Spurs and Plantar Fasciitis

A heel spur is a point of excess bone growth on the heel that usually extends forward toward the toes. Heel spurs are visible on x-rays, which is how their existence is confirmed.

The most common heel problems are actually caused by a painful tearing of the *plantar fascia* connecting the toes and the heel. This can result in either a heel spur or *plantar fasciitis*.

If your foot flattens or becomes unstable during critical times in the walking or running cycle, the attachment of the plantar fascia to your heel bone may begin to stretch and pull away. This will result in pain and possibly swelling. The pain is especially noticeable when you push off with your toes while walking, since this movement stretches the already inflamed portion of the fascia.

Without treatment, the pain will usually spread around the heel. The pain is usually centered just in front of the heel toward the arch. When the tearing occurs at the bone itself, the bone may attempt to heal itself by producing new bone. This results in the development of a heel spur. Without the spur, the condition is called plantar fasciitis.

The pain of this condition can cause you to try to walk on your toes or alter your running stride and gait, which will cause further damage and may cause a problem to develop in your healthy foot. Gait changes in running can also lead to ankle, knee, hip, or back pain.

Causes of Heel Spurs and Plantar Fasciitis

The most frequent cause of these injuries is excessive pronation. Normally, while walking or during long-distance running, your foot will strike the ground on the heel, then roll forward toward your toes and inward to the arch. Your arch should only dip slightly during this motion. If it lowers too much, you have what is known as excessive pronation. (For more details on pronation, see the section on biomechanics and gait in Chapter 13.)

The mechanical structure of your feet and the manner in which the different segments of your feet are linked together and joined with your legs has a major effect on their function and on the development of mechanically caused problems. Having badly functioning feet with poor bone alignment will adversely affect the muscles, ligaments, and tendons and can create a variety of aches and pains. Excess pronation can cause the arch of your foot to stretch excessively with each step. It can also cause too much motion in segments of the foot that should be stable as you are walking or running. This hypermobility may cause other bones to shift as well as other mechanically induced problems.

Other factors that can contribute to plantar fasciitis and heel spurs include a sudden increase in daily activities, increase in weight (not usually a problem with runners), or a change of shoes. Dramatic increase in training intensity or duration can cause plantar fasciitis.

Treatment of Plantar Fasciitis

As with most running-related injuries, evaluate any changes in your training. A decrease in workout intensity and duration is important. Self-treatment for this condition entails making sure that your shoes offer motion control and that they're not contributing to plantar fasciitis and heel spurs.

Check your running shoes to make sure they are not excessively worn. They should bend only at the ball of the foot, where your toes attach to the foot. This is vital! Avoid any shoe that bends in the center of the arch or behind the ball of the foot. It offers insufficient support and will stress your plantar fascia. The human foot was not designed to bend here, and neither should a shoe be designed to do this.

Shoe Pushup Test

Perform the shoe pushup test to check where your shoe ends. Hold the heel of the shoe in one hand and then press up underneath the forefoot (where the ball of the foot would be, forward). The shoe should bend at the ball of the shoe, where the metatarsals would be. Next, press under the part of the shoe where the metatarsal heads would be. The shoe should not bend under moderate pressure in this area.

The treatment plan that seems to work best includes carefully following a program of physical therapy with the application of felt straps to the feet. The physical therapy modalities most frequently used include ultrasound (high frequency sound vibrations that create a deep heat and reduce inflammation) and galvanic (a carefully applied intermittent muscular stimulation to the heel and calf that helps reduce pain and relax muscle spasm, which is a contributing factor to the pain). This treatment has been found most effective when given twice a week. The felt pads strapped to your feet will compress after a few days and must be reapplied. While wearing them, they should be kept dry, but they can be removed the night before your next appointment.

Following control of the pain and inflammation associated with this injury, you should use an orthotic to stabilize your foot and prevent a recurrence. More than 98 percent of the time, heel spurs and plantar fasciitis can be controlled by this treatment, and surgery can be avoided. The orthotic prevents excess pronation and prevents lengthening of the plantar fascia and continued tearing of the fascia. Usually a slight heel lift and a firm shank in the shoe will also help to reduce the severity of this problem.

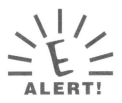
ALERT!

It is important to be aware of how your foot feels over the course of therapy. If your foot is still uncomfortable without the strapping but was more comfortable while wearing it, that is an indication that the treatment should help. Remember, what took many months or years to develop cannot be eliminated in just a few days.

Neuroma Pain

Neuroma pain is classically described as a burning pain in the forefoot. It can also be felt as an aching or shooting pain in this area. You might feel like you want to take off your shoes and rub your foot. It may occur in the middle of a run or at the end of a long run. If your shoes are quite tight, it may occur very early in the run.

Causes of Neuroma Pain

The source of this pain is an enlargement of the sheath of an intermetatarsal nerve in the foot. This usually occurs in the space between the third and fourth toes and metatarsals, which is where the intermetatarsal nerve is thickest.

Pronation of the foot can cause the metatarsal heads to rotate slightly and pinch the nerve that runs between the metatarsal heads. This chronic pinching can make the nerve sheath enlarge. As it enlarges, it becomes more squeezed and increasingly troublesome.

Treating Neuroma

Treatment of this condition is mostly practical, having a lot to do with your shoes. It includes wearing shoes with a wide toe box, not lacing the forefoot part of your shoe too tightly, and making sure your feet are in supportive shoes but not being squeezed. If this doesn't relieve the pain, work with a doctor to decide on these treatments: orthotics, an injection of steroids, or surgical removal of the neuroma, preferably in that order.

Chapter 15

Injuries of the Leg and Other Areas

Chapter 14 provided an overview of common injuries to the foot and ankle. As stated there, it is beyond the scope of this book to provide detailed information about treatments without knowing all the symptoms. Every injury is unique, and for best results, you should work with a trusted sports physician to determine the appropriate course of treatment. (See Chapter 13 for information on how to find a sports doctor.) This chapter provides an overview of injuries of the leg and other areas affected by running, listed in alphabetical order.

15

Anterior Shin Splints

The medical term *anterior shin splints* has been replaced in the past three years. Now the symptoms that occur in the anterior lateral tibial region are assumed to be either stress fractures or a form of compartment syndrome. In understanding the anterior shin splint, it is therefore important to differentiate a shin splint from a stress fracture.

Most injuries that fit the term anterior shin splint are soft tissue injuries that occur where the muscle and bone meet. These usually result in a more vertical area of symptoms.

The involved section of the upper tibia is usually five to eight centimeters long and about one to two centimeters wide. Most injuries that clinically seem to be stress fractures have what is called a region of pinpoint tenderness and extend in a horizontal direction. This line in many stress fractures of the tibia extends horizontally, but might take a tangential course through the tibia. For injuries that are horizontal, no tenderness is found one or two centimeters above or below this discrete line of tenderness.

The nonstress fracture to this area may be due to microtears of the muscle either at the origin or in the fibers themselves. This may occur because of repetitive traction or pulling of the anterior tibial muscles at their site of origin. Repetitive loading with excessive stress, such as caused by running on concrete, may also play a role in injury to this area. This can result in microtrauma to the bone structure itself.

Anterior Compartment Syndrome

One should be aware that a compartment syndrome can occur here. This is usually chronic, repetitive, and in some respects different from the acute compartment syndrome seen after serious muscle injuries. It is vital to seek evaluation and treatment if this is suspected. It is caused by the muscles swelling within a closed compartment, with a resultant increase in pressure. The blood supply can be compromised and muscle injury and pain may occur. The symptoms include leg pain, unusual nerve sensations (paresthesia), and later, muscle weakness. Definitive evaluation measures the pressure in the compartment. Surgical decompression of the compartment may be required to relieve pain.

Runners at Risk for Anterior Shin Splints

The usual runners at risk for anterior shin splints are beginning runners not yet acclimated to the stresses of running. They also may not have been doing an adequate amount of stretching. Poor choice of shoes and running surface (such as concrete) can also play a role. Overtraining, of course, can be a factor, as with most running injuries.

The usual mechanical factor seen is an imbalance between the posterior and anterior muscle groups. The posterior muscles may be both too tight and too strong. The effect of too tight posterior musculature has ramifications for the gait cycle at two points.

The first period in which too tight posterior muscles impact the anterior muscles is just before and after heel contact by the distance runner. At this time, the anterior muscles are acting as decelerators. If the posterior muscles are too tight, they force the anterior muscles to work longer and harder in this deceleration.

The second point in the gait cycle at which the anterior muscles may work too hard is when the foot leaves the ground, at toe off. The anterior muscles should be lifting up, or dorsiflexing, the foot at this time so that the toes clear the ground as the leg is brought forward. If the posterior muscles are too tight, the anterior muscles again work harder than they should. Logically, downhill running also has an adverse effect on the anterior muscles.

Repetitive impact on hard surfaces is another frequently associated factor. Excessive pronation may be a minor factor, though it is a much greater factor in medial shin splints. Overstriding during speed work in underconditioned runners can also contribute to this problem.

Self-Care

Decrease training immediately. Do not run if pain occurs during or following your run. Nonweight-bearing exercise may be necessary. Your goal is to find the distance you can run (if any) that does not produce symptoms—rather than to find your real limit. Swimming, biking, and pool running can all be used to maintain fitness. Review your stretching, and think about what good habits can keep you out of the doctor's office.

The posterior muscles should be gently stretched. (See both Chapter 7 and the stretching tips in Chapter 13.) It's recommended that you do gentle stretching of the calf muscles and the hamstrings.

Replace shoes with too many miles on them. Shock absorption should be a factor in selecting shoes if you have anterior shin splints. Downhill running can aggravate this problem and should be avoided. A stride that's too long can also delay healing. Most of all, do not run on concrete. After exercise, apply ice to lessen symptoms.

Office Medical Care of Anterior Shin Splints

A thorough evaluation of your training and racing schedule and shoes is followed by a biomechanical evaluation. A bone scan can be used, if necessary, to evaluate the possibility of stress fracture. A wick catheter test can be used, if necessary, to measure post-exercise compartment pressure, if a compartment syndrome is suspected.

Anti-inflammatory medication can be prescribed. The use of physical therapy modalities and electrical stimulation (HVGS) can also be helpful to treat this problem.

Sometimes a heel lift is used to reduce the pulling effect of tight posterior muscles. Even though this increases the distance the foot must be dorsiflexed, the duration of action and the effective strength of the posterior muscles is decreased. Orthotics may also be considered when biomechanical abnormalities exist and problems persist.

Dry Heaves or Vomiting

Dry heaves have been associated with training that goes into the anaerobic (without oxygen) realm. If you feel dry heaves coming on at the end of your interval or race, slow down but keep moving. Don't stop. The movement will help keep your heart pumping, the blood flowing, and flush out some of the lactic acid buildup. Slowing down at the end of your workout also helps your body adapt to a more static state. A proper cool-down is always in order—good for the muscles, the body, and the soul. After that, you can hydrate and jump into the shower.

Iliotibial Band (ITB) Syndrome

Symptoms of *iliotibial band syndrome* are pain or aching on the outer side of the knee. This usually happens in the middle or at the end of a run. Factors contributing to this syndrome are weak hip abductor muscles, bow legs, pronation of the foot, leg length discrepancy, and running on a crowned (convex) surface. Circular track running may also contribute to this problem since it stresses the body in a manner similar to that of crowned surfaces and leg length differences.

Anatomy of the IT Band

All of these factors are aggravated by a tight iliotibial band. The iliotibial band is a thickening of the lateral (outer) soft tissue that envelops the leg. Changes in training (often sudden increases in mileage) frequently contribute to this problem. It is always important to examine your training regimen to see what alterations have recently occurred.

Treatment for ITB Syndrome

To self-treat this problem, you should:

- Temporarily decrease training
- Side stretch
- Avoid crowned surfaces or too much running around a track
- Shorten your stride
- Wear more motion-control shoes to limit pronation
- Strengthen your hip abductor muscles (gluteus medius muscle)
- Carefully examine your training regimen (and running diary)

Side stretching is performed while standing as follows: Place your injured leg behind the good one. If the left side is the sore side, cross your left leg behind your right one. Then lean away from the injured side toward your right side. Lean on a table or chair for balance as you do this. Hold for 7–10 seconds, and repeat on each side 7–10 times. Be careful not to overstretch.

Hip abductor strengthening starts by standing on one leg with your other knee bent. You then tilt your hip and pelvis down and then lift them back up, keeping the knee straight on the leg on which you are standing.

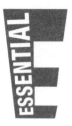

If your self-treatment is not completely successful, then a trip to a sports medicine specialist may result in either a steroid injection below the IT band or a recommendation for orthotics. Treatment is usually successful for this problem.

Medial Shin Splints (MTSS)

The outmoded term *medial shin splints* has been replaced by *medial tibial stress syndrome* (MTSS). Either term suffices to describe pain at the medial aspect of the leg, adjacent to the medial tibia. Tenderness is usually found between 3–12 centimeters above the tip of the *medial malleolus* at the posterio-medial aspect of the tibia.

When the tibia is palpated (touched), the tenderness is not directly medial but is just behind the most medial portion of the tibia, in the mass of soft tissue there and at the bone itself. Periostitis sometimes occurs in this location. The sore, inflamed structures usually include the medial muscles and tendons here. The posterior tibial tendon and muscle are frequently involved, as well as the *flexor digitorum longus* and *flexor hallucis longus*.

Stress fractures can also occur in this area. The definitive test for stress fracture is a bone scan, but false negatives can occur. It is possible that a false positive might occur also because of the soft tissue and periosteal involvement in this injury. Clinical examination is used to differentiate between medial shin splints and a stress fracture. With medial shin splints, the tenderness extends along a considerable vertical distance of the tibia. When a stress fracture is present, tenderness usually extends horizontally across the inside and front of the tibia.

Risk Factors

The first risk factor is overtraining. Evaluate your schedule to determine what training errors you may have made. Mechanically, pronation is most likely to be the culprit. When the foot pronates, the medial structures of the leg are stretched and stressed, which increases the likelihood of injury. Running on a cambered surface, such as the side of a crowned road, can put the upper leg at risk of developing this problem because the corresponding foot is functioning in a pronated position.

Treating MTSS

Decrease training immediately. Do not run if pain occurs during or following your run. Nonweight-bearing exercise may be necessary. Swimming, biking, and pool running can all be used to maintain fitness. Although running on soft surfaces has been recommended for this problem, it is not likely to help a pure MTSS. The foot is more likely to pronate excessively on mushy grass or sand. Packed dirt is ideal, and avoidance of concrete is also helpful.

In many cases, shoes rated high for control of pronation may be helpful. Gentle posterior stretching exercises may help, but control of pronation is more direct. Ice applications following running can offer some relief but are not curative. If symptoms persist, it is important to seek professional medical attention.

In the doctor's office, a thorough medical evaluation of your training schedule, racing schedule, and shoes is followed by a biomechanical evaluation. Anti-inflammatory medication can be prescribed. The use of physical therapy modalities such as electrical stimulation (HVGS) and ultrasound can also be helpful to treat this problem, as can taping the foot to limit pronation and decrease the stress on the medial structures of the leg. Pronation, which is a major contributing factor to this syndrome, can be corrected with improved shoes and over-the-counter or custom orthotics.

Runner's Knee

The knee is a complex joint. It includes the articulation between the tibia and femur (leg and thigh) and the patella (kneecap). The most common knee problems in running concern what is called the *patello-femoral complex,* comprised of the quadriceps, kneecap, and *patellar tendon.* What is called runner's knee (*Chondromalacia Patella Syndrome*) is a softening of the cartilage of the kneecap. Cartilage does not have the same blood supply that bone does.

Causes of Runner's Knee

During running, certain mechanical conditions can predispose you to a mistracking kneecap. Portions of the cartilage may then be under either too much or too little pressure, and the appropriate intermittent compression needed for waste removal and nutrition supply may not be present. This can result in cartilage deterioration, which at the knee usually occurs on the medial aspect or inner part of the kneecap.

The symptoms of runner's knee include pain near the kneecap, usually at the medial (inner) portion and below it. Pain is usually felt after sitting for a long period of time with the knees bent. Running downhill and sometimes even walking down stairs can be followed by pain. When the knee is bent, there is increased pressure between the joint surface of the kneecap and the femur (thigh bone). This stresses the injured area and leads to pain.

What is known as the *Q* (quadriceps) angle increases the chance of having runner's knee. The *Q* angle is an estimate of the effective angle at which the quadriceps averages its pull. It is determined by drawing a line from the *anterior superior iliac spine* (the bump above and in front of your hip joint) to the center of your kneecap, and a second line from the center of your kneecap to the insertion of the patellar tendon (where the tendon below your kneecap inserts). Normal is below twelve degrees, while definitely abnormal is above fifteen degrees.

Often, adding to the strong lateral pull of the bulk of the quadriceps is a weak *vastus medialis.* This is the portion of the quadriceps that helps medially to stabilize the patella. It runs along the inside portion of the thigh bone to join at the kneecap with the other three muscles making up the quadriceps. Mechanical conditions that contribute to this include:

- Wide hips (female runners)
- Knock-knees
- Unstable kneecap (*sublaxating patella*)
- High kneecap (*patella alta*)
- Weak thigh muscle
- Pronation of the feet

Treating Runner's Knee

At the early stage of runner's knee, you should decrease running to lessen stress to this area and allow healing to begin. It is important to avoid downhill running, which stresses the patello-femoral complex. Avoid performing exercises with the knee bent. When the knee is bent, the forces under the kneecap are increased. For many with runner's knee, the *vastus medialis* muscle works only during the final thirty degrees of extension of the knee. This is the muscle that helps stabilize the kneecap medially, preventing it from shifting laterally and tracking improperly at the patello-femoral joint.

Straight-leg lifts strengthen the vastus medialis and do not significantly stress the undersurface of the kneecap. Straight-leg lifts also train all of the quadriceps muscles to fire and work synergistically (at the same time). You should do these ten times on each side and repeat, beginning with five sets of ten and working your way up to ten sets of ten. Straight-leg lifts are best performed lying on a cushioned but firm surface, holding the exercising leg straight and the nonexercising leg somewhat bent to take pressure off the back.

You should stretch tight posterior muscles. In many cases, tight calf muscles or hamstrings lead to a *functional equinous* and make the foot pronate while running or walking. This pronation is accompanied by an internal rotation of the leg, which increases the Q angle and contributes to the lateral dislocation of the kneecap. You should wear running shoes that offer extra support. If you need further control of pronation, consider orthotics. Usually, trying to stretch the quadriceps itself is counterproductive. This is often done with the knee bent and puts compression forces on the undersurface of the knee cap. If you would like to stretch the quadriceps, stand near a wall and move your entire leg backward the way a ballerina does.

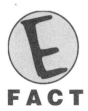

FACT

The late George Sheehan, M.D., sports medicine physician and philosopher, first popularized the practice of examining the foot when runner's knee occurs. It is also important to rule out other knee problems when knee pain occurs from running, rather than attributing every such pain to runner's knee.

Shin Splints

In the past, the medical term *shin splint* was used to diagnose almost all problems occurring in the lower leg. These included both bone and soft tissue problems and those that overlapped. Now doctors use the terms *medial tibial stress syndrome, compartment syndrome,* and *stress fracture* to describe injuries of the lower leg. These are discussed earlier in this chapter.

Defining the Problem

Most athletes refer to pain occurring either in the anterior or the medial portion of the leg as a shin splint. Problems that occur in the lateral aspect of the leg are usually either fibular stress fractures or peroneal tendon injuries following an inversion injury of the ankle. Posterior leg pains are frequently injuries to the posterior muscle group at the *myotendinous junction* of the calf muscles and Achilles tendon, or early Achilles tendonitis.

Side Stitches

Side stitches are pains that occur usually just under the ribs when running. It seems that an unconditioned diaphragm is the cause of this pain more often than not. Some other causes of this pain include food allergies (often milk), gas, or just having eaten before running. Also, running a greater distance or at a faster pace than usual will bring this on. Side stitches seem to occur most often on the right side of the body. It is possible that the liver alters the motion of the diaphragm more on that side because of the larger right lobe.

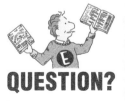

QUESTION?

What is a diaphragm?
The diaphragm is a muscle that separates the chest cavity from the abdomen. It moves down when you inhale and moves up when you exhale. When subject to increased or faster exercise than it is accustomed to, it can cramp and cause pain.

Controlling Side Stitches

When caused by lack of conditioning, the best thing to do for side stitches is to run slower and longer. Breathe fuller and try belly breathing, in which you allow your stomach to relax and push out as you inhale and then contract slightly as you exhale fully. Breathe rhythmically and make sure that you are not holding your breath.

Another breathing tactic consists of exhaling against resistance through pursed lips. Combined with belly breathing, this may be the best approach. To further strengthen your diaphragm, add abdominal exercises to your regimen. Another way of gaining temporary relief is to stretch your arms up while inhaling, imagining your breath coming in and soothing the side stitch.

Chapter 16

All about Nutrition

Nutrition is one of the most important considerations you face as a runner, especially as you begin
to build toward longer runs and marathons. Eating
right is a major contributor to your overall comfort
level and enhanced performance. The information
in this chapter will keep you up to date with current medical thinking regarding sports nutrition.

Preventive Medicine

Preventive medicine holds that if you take steps to avoid injury, it is less likely to occur. Another preventive measure is to provide for your body from the inside out: Feed your body what it needs to work to capacity, and it will be better able to perform. To that end, nutritional therapy can help. This includes:

- A regular source of high-quality protein as part of your meals.
- Vitamin C to support healing, reduce swelling, repair tissue, and keep ligaments and tendons strong.
- Calcium and magnesium as essential for bone and muscle health.
- Bromelain to help reduce swelling, especially when taken with turmeric.
- Zinc as important for bone health and tissue repair.
- Omega-3 fatty acids, such as flax and fish oils, as natural anti-inflammatories.

A Nutritious Mindset

What to eat, when to eat, even how to eat—all of this you learn from your parents and peers. Really, it's not until you're a teenager that you have much of a choice about what you eat. And then it becomes fun to eat all the "bad" stuff—fast food, high-fat snacks, pizza with extra, extra cheese. It's easy and gratifying to include these foods as part of your regular meals. So, of course, they become habits—habits that lead to weight gain, lethargy, and even addiction.

When a Diet Isn't a Diet

A diet is actually made up of the foods you live on day after day. It doesn't matter whether you eat poorly or well; your diet consists of the foods you consume. Period. In the United States, though, diet has come to mean what you're restricted to eat in order to lose weight. Because most Americans have been on diets and certainly exposed to the diet culture, it's hard for them not to associate diet with tough choices, overconscientious eating, and, ultimately, frustration.

So one habit you have to mentally overcome is thinking of your diet as a faddish weight-loss plan. Instead, envision your diet as the fuel that feeds your machine (your body). Do you want to keep filling up your tank with crud that ultimately leads to breakdowns, or do you want to take in the kind of fuel that keeps your system running at its very best and that guarantees performance? If you're reading this book and are serious about your fitness and training, you undoubtedly will choose the latter.

Nutrition Know-How

To get the most out of the fuel you put into your body, you have to understand what makes up the fuel. What is in the fuel that provides energy? What is in the fuel that is wasteful or harmful? What is the right balance of nutrients that help you feel your best? What nutritionists, doctors, and scientists have found optimal is a meal that breaks out thus: 55–60 percent of total calories from carbohydrates, 25 percent from fat, and 15 percent from protein. These are three of the six essential nutrients your body needs. The others are water, vitamins, and minerals. All are discussed in this chapter.

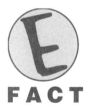

FACT

The chemical processes in your body that break down and synthesize nutrients in food are called your *metabolism.* Everyone's metabolism is different, which is why some people can seemingly eat anything and never gain weight while others need to constantly monitor the amount they eat.

Carbohydrates

A simplified way to think of carbohydrates is with this rhyme: Carbohydrates come from the ground, proteins run around. This means carbohydrates are typically found in grains, fruits, and vegetables (and proteins typically in meats). In reality, it's more complicated than that. Carbohydrates are actually the sugars, starches, and cellulose the body needs for energy. They come in two forms: complex carbohydrates and simple carbohydrates.

Complex Carbohydrates

Complex carbohydrates are what are most commonly referred to as *carbs.* Chemically more complex than simple carbohydrates, they also take longer to break down and enter the bloodstream. They are higher in fiber and lower in fat and calories than simple carbohydrates, and they last longer, giving the body energy over a longer period of time. The body stores complex carbohydrates in the liver and muscles as glycogen.

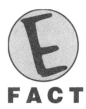

FACT

Complex carbohydrates are found in vegetables, beans, grain, and pasta. Some high-quality complex carbohydrates are brown rice, whole grains, broccoli, dried peas, beans and lentils, corn, bananas and other fresh and dried fruits, pumpkin, sweet potatoes—and, of course, pasta.

Simple Carbohydrates

Simple carbohydrates are the ones that give you instant energy. Their molecular structure is simpler than their complex counterparts, so their energy gets into your system quite rapidly. They also have a shorter lifespan and are typically lower in fiber and higher in calories. Common simple carbohydrates are found in processed sugar and other processed foods, and some fruits. Examples include white bread, potato chips, fried rice, and sweetened cereals.

Fats

If there's a nutrient with a bad rap, it's fat. But notice, fat should make up a slightly greater percentage of your daily food than protein! That's because fat supplies essential fatty acids, which furnish energy for aerobic activities like walking and climbing stairs. Stored fat insulates vital organs and transports fat-soluble vitamins (A, D, E, and K). Fat actually can be your friend. Like carbohydrates, there are also two kinds of fat: saturated and unsaturated.

Saturated Fats

Saturated fats are the "bad" kind—those that block your arteries and don't make much of a contribution to your overall health. You still need some of them, but not much; restrict them to about 10 percent of your total calories (less than one-third of your total fat intake). You'll find saturated fats in whole dairy products such as butter, cheese, and ice cream; coconut, cottonseed, and palm kernel oils; and in beef, pork, ham, and sausage.

Unsaturated Fats

Unsaturated fats come in two varieties: monounsaturated and polyunsaturated. Monounsaturated fats are found in olive and canola oils, whereas corn, safflower, soybean, and sunflower oils all contain polyunsaturated fats.

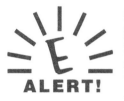

ALERT!

Otherwise known as hydrogenated vegetable oils, trans fatty acids (TFAs) are recognized and used by the body as saturated fats. Hydrogenation is the process of adding hydrogen to polyunsaturated fats to give foods a longer shelf life and added flavor. TFAs are found in commercial cookies, crackers, and fried foods.

Protein

Considered the building block of all tissues and cells, protein's primary function is to build and repair red blood cells, muscle, hair, and cells for body tissues. Protein is a secondary energy provider (to carbohydrates). It's in meat, fish, dairy products like cheese, milk, and yogurt, and in the edible parts of leguminous plants like beans, peas, and lentils.

Water

You could survive for many days without food, but without water you would die more rapidly. The human body is 60–70 percent water, which needs to be replenished constantly. Water is responsible for transporting nutrients, gases, and waste products, and for regulating your body's temperature. It is not only vitally necessary for good health, it has side benefits of being able to cool or heat your body as well as moisturize and soothe your insides (and skin). It can also help you feel full and curb your appetite.

Drinking Enough Water

It was once thought that there was no limit to the amount of water you could drink in a day, but recently there have been alarming cases of hyponatremia—of drinking too much water. That said, chances are slight that you will drink enough water in a day to experience this. Most people drink well under the recommended daily amount of water for adults, which is sixty-four ounces. The truth is, most people don't drink enough water. They're more accustomed to drinking soda, juice, coffee, tea, and alcohol. How often have you heard that you'll feel better just by taking in your sixty-four ounces of water every day? Well, it's true.

Hydrating Versus Dehydrating Fluids

You could argue that since many beverages are made with water, they should count toward your daily sixty-four ounces. This depends on the type of beverage. Hydrating beverages, all of which contribute to an improved functioning of your body, include (besides water) sports drinks that replace electrolytes; fruit juices (the less sugar, the better); soy or rice beverages (good whole milk replacements); herbal teas; and milk.

It doesn't help to cheat here, though. Milk may be hydrating, for example, but it's not a good idea to drink much more than sixteen ounces of it a day, particularly if whole milk. And although juices do contain fruit, most readily available juices have sugar as their main ingredient (a simple carb that will lift you up and drop you down).

Dehydrating fluids contain water, but they also rob your body of water. These are caffeinated and alcoholic beverages. To minimize their effect, drink water with them in a 1:1 ratio.

Vitamins and Minerals

There's a vitamin for practically every letter in the alphabet, even a few with the same letter. Why are there so many vitamins? Because vitamins perform a lot of functions in the body. For example, vitamin A is a moisturizer for your skin and mucous membranes and also aids vision. Meanwhile, vitamin C is responsible for intracellular maintenance of bone, capillaries, and teeth, and vitamin E protects polyunsaturated fats and prevents cell membrane damage.

Simplify your thinking about vitamins by remembering that the best way to get essential vitamins is through your food. So if you're eating right (according to your size, degree of stress, and exercise-level requirements), chances are you're getting most of the vitamins you need. With our demanding lifestyles and reliance on more packaged and processed foods, however, vitamin supplements can be helpful.

Some Supplements to Consider

Minerals like vitamins are necessary to aid and induce a number of vital bodily functions.

- Vitamin C supports healing, reduces swelling, repairs tissue, and keeps ligaments and tendons strong.
- Vitamin B2, or riboflavin, assists in the breakdown of carbohydrates and fats to provide energy for working muscles.
- Calcium aids in building strong bones, teeth, blood clotting, and nerve and muscle function.
- Magnesium aids in bone growth as well as nerve, muscle, and enzyme function.
- Bromelain helps reduce swelling, especially when taken with turmeric.

- Zinc is important for bone health and tissue repair.
- Phosphorous aids in the development of bones, teeth, and energy transfer.
- Omega-3 fatty acids, such as flax or fish oils, are natural anti-inflammatories.

Unfortunately, eating a healthy diet is not as easy as taking a lot of supplements. In fact, overdoing any minerals or vitamins can be dangerous, disrupting your body's balance in any of these areas.

Fiber and Cholesterol

Fiber and cholesterol are other substances contributing nutritionally to your overall health that aren't included in the Big Six.

Fiber is an essential aid in healthy digestion that cannot itself be digested. It is the roughage that passes through your system, attracting and absorbing water, digested food, and cholesterol. The source of fiber is the plant cell walls, which are broken down considerably during the processing of food. There are two types of fiber, soluble and insoluble, and the recommended daily allowance is about thirty grams combined.

Insoluble fiber attracts water and digested food; soluble fiber goes the extra mile and also attracts cholesterol. Fiber-rich foods include whole grains, fruits, and vegetables. Drinking lots of water also helps fiber do its job.

Cholesterol

Like discussions about fat, those about cholesterol are usually negative. Excess cholesterol sticks to the walls of your arteries, causing blockage. The source of cholesterol is animal-based food products: meat, fish, poultry, eggs, and dairy products.

However, cholesterol is important to health. It aids in the synthesis of adrenal (kidney) and sex hormones, vitamin D, and bile. Cholesterol is naturally produced in the liver. The Food and Drug Administration (FDA) recommends consuming less than 300 milligrams per day of cholesterol.

Here's how the cholesterol stacks up in some common foods:

- 1 ground beef patty (medium-sized): 74 mg
- 1 cup shredded cheddar cheese: 119 mg
- 1 hardboiled or poached egg: 212 mg (all from the yolk)
- 1 cup ice cream: up to 290 mg

Eating Right for Running

Now it's time to learn how to turn nutrition knowledge into sound food choices that enable you to perform at an optimal level while feeling better overall. Remember, diet is not just about losing weight, it's about properly fueling the daily activities you undertake so that you can fully participate in and enjoy them.

It Starts in the Brain

How do you know when you're hungry? Does your stomach grumble? Perhaps. Do you feel distracted, as if you're waiting for something to happen? Probably. Have you been so hungry sometimes that you feel like you could eat almost anything? So hungry that you become impatient waiting or looking for something to eat? When you have any of these sensations, it means your brain is glucose-deprived.

When your brain doesn't get the fuel it needs, besides making you feel ravenous, it can also make you feel shaky, irritable, indecisive, sluggish, and headachy. A part of your subconscious mind takes over and sends out survival signals to eat. This typically leads to poor nutritional choices, whether because you wolf down nutrient-poor snacks or junk food or because you eat too much too quickly.

Satisfying Your Mind and Your Body

To supply your body with the energy it needs, you need to be aware of three things:

1. The types of food and beverages you are consuming
2. The amounts you are eating and drinking
3. The timing, or when you are eating and drinking

What you need is a basic plan about how to eat so these three requirements are met and your body has what it needs to maximize energy and achieve metabolic maintenance. This is particularly important for you as a runner because, like a car heading out on a long trip, you need all your fluids topped to operate in your best form.

Pace and Calories

It has been estimated that between 100–120 calories are burned per mile. This rate appears to be fairly constant and independent of running speed. Although there is a slight increase in the rate of calorie burning with an increase in speed, it is considered negligible. One of the obvious advantages of running, when it comes to burning calories, is the shorter time it takes to burn the same number of calories compared with walking, bicycling, swimming, and most other aerobic exercises. Many physiologists also believe that your metabolic rate remains higher for several hours after exercise. Runners often notice a decrease in appetite after a good run. On the other hand, with this increased burning of calories, more food can safely be enjoyed!

How to Eat Right

Studies have shown that the most effective way to feed your body is by eating breakfast, snacking, eating 2–3 hours before going to sleep, and manipulating your fat-cell storage.

Eating Breakfast

Even after a mere 4–5 hours of sleep, when you awake in the morning your body is coming out of a fasting period. The fuel tank is on low or empty. Even if you don't feel hungry in the morning, it's important to "break the fast" and replenish nutrients. This prevents your brain from sending out hunger-alert signals later in the morning and stabilizes your energy needs for later in the day. Psychologically, having something to eat in the morning prevents you from feeling like you can overindulge later to make up for the skipped meal.

Snacking

If you were raised to refrain from snacking because it ruined your appetite for main meals, snacking is a tough habit to adopt. If you are a snacker already but feel you are overweight, you may want to examine the types of snacks you're eating and when you're eating them. Let's be clear: A snack is a small amount of food eaten between meals whose purpose is to prevent blood-sugar levels from dropping too low. The best snacks are those made up of complex carbohydrates that are low in fat and high in fiber, such as fruit, whole grains, and some vegetables.

Also referred to as grazing, snacking is actually the preferred way to eat. Rather than consuming three large meals (breakfast, lunch, and dinner), grazing means spreading your total caloric intake throughout the day, eating smaller yet satisfying portions of food every three or so hours.

Getting into the habit of snacking means breaking the habit of only eating at regular meal times. Unfortunately, if you're part of the working world built around regularly scheduled eating times, that can be hard to do. Many managers don't take too kindly to seeing people snack at their desks, and in some jobs there is simply no time between meals to manage to eat at all. If you haven't eaten breakfast before arriving at work, your only opportunity to eat may not come until your scheduled lunch break.

In situations like these, there is usually still time to ingest a fluid—water, coffee, juice, or soda. If so, experiment with nutritional shakes and drinks. Many are designed for people who tend to skip meals and provide the nutrients of a well-balanced meal. There are also drinkable yogurts and fruit and vegetable juices that meet many of your nutritional needs. These include carrot juice, low-sodium canned vegetable juice, pomegranate juice, and other juices that do not contain high-fructose corn syrup.

Healthy Grazing

Fruits and vegetables top the list of healthy grazing foods, and items like sliced apples or oranges, bananas, seedless grapes, peaches, pears, and plums are easy to pack for on-the-go eating. There are also many pre-washed vegetables on the market now that make snacking simple. These include baby carrots, celery slices, a combination of lettuces, snow peas, and many others. Put some all-natural peanut or almond butter on the celery slices, or make a tea sandwich out of whole grain bread spread with nut butter and topped with a sliced banana. Another great sandwich that can be cut into small pieces for easy munching is whole grain pita with hummus and greens such as broccoli slaw. Lots of cheeses (like cheddar, brie, or herbed goat cheese) go well with apples, pears, and grapes. Then there's always microwave popcorn (a "lite" variety is best) or a serving of healthy breakfast cereal chased by an organic, low-fat yogurt.

Eating Long Before Going to Sleep

After you eat, your body gets busy processing its food. This is called digestion. The body also has a long to-do list during the time that you're asleep. If the body needs both to digest and to tackle its to-do list at the same time (meaning you've eaten just before going to sleep), it's not going to be able to do its best work. It's like your boss giving you an extra assignment just as you're about to quit for the day. Make every effort to eat a small, healthy snack 2–3 hours before you go to sleep if you want your body to process the food optimally.

Eating for the Early Morning Runner

For many people, the best time to run is when they first get up in the morning, before the commitments of family and work. In light of this discussion about how important it is to break the night's fast and have enough fuel for the day, are runners who work out before breakfast ultimately causing their bodies to store fat?

In general, getting a run in before breakfast is fine so long as you aren't skipping breakfast all together. Optimally, you want to ingest some form of complex carbohydrate and fluid before you set off. A big glass of orange juice (with pulp) along with a glass of water helps. Following your run and 5–10 minutes of stretching, when you've cooled off, have a bagel, whole grain bread or cereal, some fruit, and lots of water for breakfast.

Getting into Eating

Now that you have an understanding of nutrition and know that you need to graze at intervals throughout the day, it's time to get to the heart of the matter: what to eat and in what quantities.

On the premise that food is energy, how much energy you expend determines how much food you should eat. This is called your daily caloric need, which can change daily depending on what comes up in your life (for example, longer runs = greater energy needs; more stress = greater energy needs; more sedentary lifestyle = fewer energy needs).

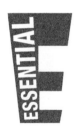

Don't forget to eat smart when dining out. Many of today's fast-food restaurants have some healthy options on their menus, and in most restaurants you can ask for salad dressing, butter, and sour cream on the side so that you can control the portions of these high-fat condiments. Ask for chicken or fish entrées broiled rather than fried. When perusing restaurant menus that offer lots of high-fat food options, make sound nutritional choices.

The first thing to do is to create an objective nutritional analysis for yourself to assess your eating habits. Since this book can't answer all your dietary questions, consult books on the subject of nutrition or ask your doctor to refer you to a nutritionist. This chapter lays the groundwork for you.

Your Eating Habits

Do you even know how much and when you eat during a typical day? Most people don't. The best way to learn is to keep a food journal for at least a week. Using a notebook, your Palm Pilot, your running log, or a calendar (something you can keep a record in), begin to write down everything you eat and when you eat it. Don't cheat! You must list even the breath mints you chew on during meetings. It's also helpful to note where your eating has taken place. At your desk? In the cafeteria? In front of the TV?

After a full week you'll have a good idea of the what, when, and where of your eating patterns. From the brief discussion here, you should be able to see from your food diary where you're making your nutritional no-noes. How often have you skipped breakfast? How often have you eaten high-fat foods like junk food, desserts, and fried food? What are your snacking habits? How many fruits and vegetables do you eat in a typical week?

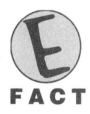

FACT

Part of eating right means counting calories, and you've been conditioned to believe that the average adult should consume no more than 2,000 calories a day. But anyone running 20–25 miles per week probably needs at least 2,500 calories a day in order to maintain adequate supplies of muscle glycogen. Being able to increase overall calorie (and carb) intake wisely is something that runners are able to enjoy.

Fat-Cell Storage

Irregular eating causes your brain to protect your fat cells, because those are what hold energy. If you have a track record of skipping meals and eating erratically, you've trained your body to store fat, which is why it might be difficult for you to lose weight. Eating regularly and healthfully means your brain doesn't have to worry about energy sources so your fat cells won't be stored—the fat in your body is used as it's needed.

Where You Are Versus Where You Need to Be

To make intelligent food choice easier, the U.S. government has formulated dietary guidelines as recommended by the American Dietetic Association, American Cancer Society, American College of Sports Medicine, American Heart Association, and the surgeon general. The recommendation is that your intake at every meal should be comprised of 55–60 percent carbohydrates, 20–30 percent fat (no more than 10 percent from saturated fat), and 10–15 percent protein. This is the balanced diet that works best to fuel your system.

Looking at these guidelines makes meal planning easier. Endurance athletes often push their carbohydrate intake to 65 percent while offsetting this by reducing their total fat calories. Applying calorie recommendations to your plate, the section for carbs should be the largest, protein next, and fat smallest (because even though the percentage of recommended fats is higher than the percentage of protein, fats have a higher caloric value).

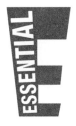

Using these U.S. government recommendations, look back at your food log for the week, charting your main meals by whether they were largely composed of carbs, protein, or fat. Surprised? Apply these recommendations at restaurants and while grocery shopping. Are meats and ice cream taking up more room than fresh vegetables, whole grains, and fresh fruit?

As a runner, you will find this nutritional information especially valuable. To eat right for running, you need the nutrients that best fuel your energy. These are carbohydrates. But proteins are essential for the utilization of energy, and fat is essential for overall good health. Consider this chapter your introduction to nutrition and healthy eating.

Chapter 17

Are You Ready for the Marathon?

The marathon is one of the most grueling events in all of organized sports. It requires long months of painstaking training and planning. Finishing a marathon is one of the most rewarding experiences any runner can possibly imagine. It takes dedication, resolve, and persistence. It is also something that should only be attempted by a runner who has some miles under her belt. Just as properly training to run a marathon and then completing one can be a highlight of your life, not training properly can leave you with not only a very bad experience but with injuries that may be difficult to overcome. If you're going to run a marathon, do it right—it's worth every minute of training.

A Brief History of the Marathon

There is probably no sporting event in the world that has more history tied to it than the marathon. It is legendary. In a nutshell, the king of the Persian Empire in the fifth century B.C. wanted to conquer Greece so he could bring his armies into Europe by land. Knowing they would be outnumbered, the Atheneans sent a foot messenger to Sparta, 150 miles away, seeking assistance to fight the Persians. That messenger was Pheidippides. He covered the distance in two days, and the Spartans were able to help the Atheneans beat back the Persian army and secure Greece. The marathon was named for the site of the battle of Marathon, approximately 25 miles from Athens, where the victory occurred.

When did the marathon become 26.2 miles? As travel writer Paul Smaras notes, "At the 1908 Olympic Games in London, the marathon distance was changed to 26 miles to cover the ground from Windsor Castle to White City stadium, with 385 yards added on so the race could finish in front of the royal family's viewing box.... After sixteen years of extremely heated discussion, this 26.2 mile distance was established at the 1924 Olympics in Paris as the official marathon distance."

Getting Down to Business: The Long Run

You should not attempt a marathon unless you have been running for at least one year and are comfortably running 25 miles a week or more. If you find that running 25 miles per week is difficult to accomplish for any number of reasons (aches and pains, time constraints, etc.), you are not yet ready to begin training for this event.

Runners training to compete in a marathon must slowly and systematically build the distance of their long runs to a minimum of 20 miles. In fact, completing three runs of 20–23 miles each in the ten weeks prior to the marathon is a realistic predictor of successfully completing the race.

Definition and Purposes of the Long Run

For the purpose of this discussion, the distance of a long run is 10 miles or longer (or a run that lasts over 90 minutes). It should be run approximately 1 minute slower than the time at which you plan to run the marathon. If your training schedule calls for a long run of 18 miles, you must run the distance at one session rather than splitting it into a 9-mile morning run and a 9-mile evening run.

The long run is the most important component of marathon training because it teaches the body both to mentally and physically tackle the challenge of completing the 26.2-mile event. Physiologically, the body must learn to draw on fat storage energy reserves after depleting glycogen fuel stores in the muscles (converted from carbohydrate food sources). You must become accustomed to running for very long periods of time. The mental toughness you develop from completing long training runs pays handsome dividends when you run the actual marathon.

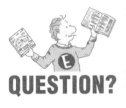

QUESTION?

What are the benefits of the long run?
The long run strengthens the heart; it strengthens the leg muscles critical for endurance; it develops mental toughness and coping skills; it increases fat-burning capacity as well as capillary growth and myoglobin concentration in muscle fibers; and it increases aerobic efficiency.

Above all, design your marathon training schedule so that you are rested prior to undertaking your long runs. If you complete two to three long training runs each of 20 miles or longer, you will no doubt reduce the possibility of hitting the dreaded "wall" during the marathon. The wall refers to the point in time during a marathon when the glycogen stores in your leg muscles become depleted, after which your pace can slow to a crawl.

The majority of runners who experience difficulty completing long training runs fail to prepare adequately for these critical workouts. So remember, neither long runs nor the marathon itself have to be painful experiences. The key is to plan ahead.

Making the Long Run Easier and Safer

Don't schedule long runs too early in your training, even if you are physically prepared to cover the distance. This can lead to staleness or premature burnout. Additionally, you could peak too early in your training. Also, schedule some long runs at the same time of day the actual marathon will be held to familiarize yourself with running during that time frame and also to develop a pre-race routine you feel comfortable with.

Consider running for cumulative time, approximating the distance (as discussed in Chapter 5). Doing so gives you more flexibility and spontaneity regarding the route you will be running. However, do your longest run no closer than three to four weeks before the marathon. The distance of this run should be 23 miles maximum. Above all, do not run 26.2 miles in practice to see if you can run a marathon. Save your efforts for the actual race!

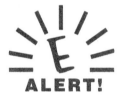

ALERT!

It is important to follow the hard-easy method of training emphasized throughout this book. Pressing too hard without scheduled rest periods or reduced workloads more often than not leads to injuries and training delays. Do not become obsessed with your training to the extent that you run on rest days. This approach can lead to injury, fatigue, and even burnout.

Do not increase the distance of your long run by more than 10 percent per week. This equates to adding approximately 15 minutes to each subsequent long run. Every fourth week (as indicated in **TABLES 17-1** and **17-2**), drop the distance of your long run along with your total weekly mileage to incorporate a light period of training. This facilitates rest and recovery.

Areas of Experimentation

One benefit of marathon training is the opportunity to experiment with various concerns (for example, shoes, nutrition) prior to incorporating practices in the actual 26.2-mile event. A cardinal rule of marathoning is:

Don't try anything new on race day. Use all training runs as an occasion for experimentation.

First, think about your shoes. If your shoes are currently causing you any discomfort during training, you should not wear them in the marathon. As soon as possible, talk to a local professional at a specialty running store for advice on a different shoe to train and race in. At least six weeks prior to the marathon, you should decide on a specific brand to wear for your final long training run and, of course, for the marathon.

Socks are also important. Which type of socks (for example, thin, thick, two layers, synthetic-blend) work best for you? There's no worse feeling in a marathon than developing blisters from your socks at only the halfway point!

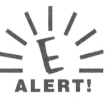
ALERT!

When training, think about running with others. Running with a group makes the long run more pleasurable and easier to accomplish than running alone. However, in running with a group, be sure you don't turn long runs into races. This will almost surely lead to injury.

Additionally, consider all of your running apparel. What type of clothing won't cause chafing? How much and what type of clothing do you need to wear to be comfortable yet not overheated (for example, gloves, hat, long sleeves)?

Beyond apparel, consider running accessories. For instance, do you plan to use analgesic creams (Ben Gay, Myoflex, Sportscreme, etc.) during the marathon? Some experts claim that these don't penetrate deeply enough to relieve muscular discomfort. Others say that creams are effective in reducing pain and inflammation. Similarly, what about a moisturizing lubricant for your skin, such as Vaseline? If you use these products, how much and where should they be applied (for example, under arms, on toes, between legs, nipples)?

For your pre-race routine, consider what you are going to eat and your pre-race evening meal. What type of high-carbohydrate meal do you crave (for example, pasta, potatoes, rice)? Which foods give you the most energy?

How much do you need to eat? Are there any foods that you should avoid so as not to cause digestive problems?

Similarly, how about the race-morning snack? What type of foods work best for you, yielding energy while not causing stomach discomfort or cramps? Should you partake of caffeine? If yes, how much should you drink and how soon before the marathon? Some research suggests that drinking caffeinated products spares glycogen early in a marathon. The downside is that caffeine is a diuretic and thus can lead to dehydration. The bottom line is that if you consume caffeine, be sure also to drink water to avoid dehydration.

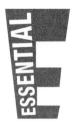

Many honey makers and produce stores sell honey sticks, plastic straws filled with flavored honeys. These are very easy to carry with you on long runs since they're small and lightweight, and they provide a safe and natural source of sugar to boost your energy.

Rest is as important as eating before a race. Figure out what time you need to retire to get a good night's sleep. Also, determine how early you need to rise to take care of needs, such as eating breakfast, hydrating, and visiting the bathroom.

During the race, you need a plan for hydration. How often do you need to drink during the marathon, and should you consume sports drinks or just water at every aid station? These are very important questions you need to decide prior to your marathon.

Finally, decide whether or not you will rely on gels as a supplemental energy source during the marathon (as many runners do). There are many types of gels to choose from nowadays. The key is finding the particular product that works for you. Training runs present opportunities to decide how many packets you will need to consume during the marathon, when to take them (at which mile markers or elapsed marathon time), along with determining whether they cause stomach discomfort.

Marathon Training Schedules

Before choosing one of the two marathon training schedules that follow, it is essential that you successfully complete a base-building period by following one of the two mileage buildup schedules outlined in Chapter 5. It cannot be stressed enough that both of the marathon training schedules offered below are designed for runners who have successfully completed the mileage buildup period. If you have not fully completed the buildup phase, then do not proceed.

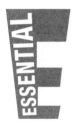

It is perfectly acceptable during a long run to come to a complete stop for 1–2 minutes to drink fluids, stretch, hit the restroom, etc. Such brief stops will have no adverse effect on your preparedness to successfully complete the marathon.

Additionally, it is crucial that you have applied the training principles and injury prevention strategies emphasized throughout this book. Using a training schedule without such basic knowledge or without the consultation of a coach or the advice of a knowledgeable and experienced runner is indeed hazardous to your health.

If you cannot complete the mileage specified for the first four weeks in these schedules without injury or resultant pain, then you should continue to work through the mileage buildup schedules. Scale back your training to a level that enables you to train safely without leg fatigue, soreness, or injury.

Schedule 1 (Beginner)

Although this schedule features a bit less weekly mileage than the advanced marathon schedule that follows (Schedule 2), runners who complete the workouts specified here will still be well-prepared to run 26.2 miles successfully on marathon day. Another attractive feature of this schedule is that it is based on a four-day training week, ideal for people faced with the demands of a busy work schedule, family commitments, and other obligations and responsibilities.

Schedule 2 (Advanced)

This is an 18-week program geared to the runner who has completed the more advanced mileage buildup schedule featuring higher weekly mileage. As with the beginner's marathon training schedule, you'll notice that this schedule builds up mileage gradually. In the first week you will run 34 miles total. You will gradually hit varying peaks in weeks 6, 11, and 14.

Table 17-1

Marathon Training Schedule 1 (Beginner)

Week	Sun.	Mon.	Tues.	Wed.	Thur.	Fri.	Sat.	Total
1	10	Rest	5	Rest	5	Rest	4	24
2	5	Rest	4	Rest	4	Rest	4	17 Light Week
3	11	Rest	5	Rest	6	Rest	4	26
4	12	Rest	6	Rest	6	Rest	4	28
5	13	Rest	6	Rest	7	Rest	4	30
6	6	Rest	4	Rest	4	Rest	4	18 Light Week
7	15	Rest	7	Rest	7	Rest	4	33
8	17	Rest	7	Rest	8	Rest	4	36
9	19	Rest	7	Rest	9	Rest	4	39
10	7	Rest	4	Rest	4	Rest	4	19 Light Week
11	221	Rest	7	Rest	9	Rest	4	41
12	14	Rest	7	Rest	10	Rest	4	35
13	8	Rest	4	Rest	4	Rest	4	20 Light Week
14	22	Rest	7	Rest	9	Rest	4	42
15	12	Rest	7	Rest	10	Rest	4	33
16	14	Rest	7	Rest	5	Rest	4	30
17	10	Rest	6	Rest	4	Rest	Rest	20 Light Week
18	26.2 Marathon	Rest	Rest	Rest	Rest	Rest	Rest	Marathon Week

Numbers refer to miles of running

Table 17-2

Marathon Training Schedule 2 (Advanced)

Week #	Sun.	Mon.	Tues.	Wed.	Thur.	Fri.	Sat.	Total
1	10	Rest	6	8	6	Rest	4	34
2	12	Rest	6	8	6	Rest	4	36
3	6	Rest	4	Rest	4	Rest	4	18 Light Week
4	14	Rest	6	8	6	Rest	4	38
5	16	Rest	6	8	6	Rest	5	41
6	18	Rest	6	8	6	Rest	5	43
7	6	Rest	5	Rest	5	Rest	4	20 Light Week
8	20	Rest	5	7	6	Rest	4	42
9	14	Rest	6	8	6	Rest	4	38
10	7	Rest	5	Rest	6	Rest	4	22 Light Week
11	21	Rest	5	7	6	Rest	4	43
12	14	Rest	6	8	6	Rest	4	38
13	8	Rest	6	Rest	6	Rest	4	24 Light Week
14	22–23	Rest	5	7	6	Rest	5	45–46
15	12	Rest	6	8	6	Rest	4	36
16	14	Rest	7	Rest	5	Rest	4	30
17	10	Rest	6	Rest	4	Rest	1–2 Optional	20–22 Taper Week
18	26.2 Marathon	Rest	Rest	Rest	Rest	Rest	Rest	Marathon Week

Numbers refer to miles of running

Mentally Training for the Marathon

This section discusses a variety of mental training strategies for the marathon. These enable you to set realistic goals, complete the necessary physical training (in particular, the long runs), and be prepared mentally for the challenges ahead.

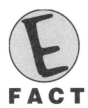

FACT

Techniques you can use to psyche yourself up during both marathon training and the actual race include mental rehearsal or visualization (creating scenarios in your mind), guided imagery (imagining how you wish an event to occur), and self-talk (giving yourself positive affirmations).

Before You Begin

There are certain mental characteristics that a runner must possess in order to undertake the necessary training that a marathon requires. These include motivation, self-discipline, and effective time management, all of which are interrelated. Although a coach can provoke interest and enthusiasm in a training program, you must develop motivation and discipline primarily within yourself.

Set Your Goals

In order to run a marathon, you need two overarching goals to motivate and sustain you. These divide into process goals and outcome goals.

Process goals focus on mastering a task and increasing your skill level. Examples of process goals include following a training schedule as closely as possible; improving your nutrition; reading as much as you can about training principles; consulting with your coach regularly; getting increased sleep to be as rested as possible; maintaining your running journal; and making sure your shoes aren't too worn.

Outcome goals relate to the finished product or, stated differently, goals you hope to accomplish in the marathon. Examples include breaking 40 minutes after running 10K; running the second half of the marathon faster than the first 13.1 miles; defeating a rival; and running a personal best in your favorite local race.

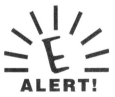
ALERT!

When setting goals, it is best to be as specific as possible. Be sure to write your goals down, not only in your running journal but, say, on an index card left in a visible place, like on your kitchen counter. This practical strategy will help you to achieve both short- and long-term marathon goals.

There are factors to take into consideration in order to create meaningful goals for yourself in a marathon. These include:

- **Timing (present life situation).** Be sure that this is a good time in your life to pursue a marathon goal. For example, if you are relocating to take a job in another city, it might be best to wait until you settle in before training for a marathon.
- **Training information.** Take a look at two or three additional sources of credible training information to understand the commitment (of time and effort) needed to achieve your marathon goal. Books, magazine articles, and Internet sites feature a variety of marathon training programs.
- **Enjoy the journey.** First and foremost, make sure your marathon goal is something you enjoy working toward and accomplishing. If you are contemplating training for a marathon but don't enjoy running more than 30 minutes at a time, you won't enjoy training for 2–3 hours at a time over the course of many weekends.
- **Enjoy the destination.** Is the outcome of your marathon goal something you would enjoy? Is the payoff worth your time and effort? Running for a charitable cause, fulfilling a life dream and earning a medal, or traveling to a beautiful destination to run a marathon with friends can be powerful motivators to see your goal through to completion.

- **Necessary weekly training time.** Be sure that you have adequate time to train during the course of the week, based on your training schedule. Be aware of the time commitment necessary to achieve your marathon goal.

- **Necessary long-term training time.** Prior to setting a marathon goal, be sure you have adequate time for long-term training. Look at the miles or minutes you are currently running when considering the feasibility of running a marathon.

- **Natural ability.** Unfortunately, not everyone is born to develop into a world-class athlete. Improvement comes quickly and relatively easily in the beginning of training, but progress doesn't come nearly as rapidly after months and years of hard work. The natural ability you are born with plays a significant role in determining your marathon outcome.

- **Be sure the goal is yours.** Just because Joe down the street is training for a marathon and has urged you to join him doesn't mean you should send off your application, too. In other words, don't get swept up emotionally and commit to a marathon goal without thinking it through.

- **Establish short-term goals leading to the big goal.** If you wish to run a marathon six months from now, then set some short-term goals along the way to keep motivated. Although it's okay to think about where you want to be years from now, focus on realizing short-term goals within a period of six months. At the same time, you can't train hard for more than three or four months at a time. Allow breaks after attaining short-term goals or peak events during your training.

- **Congruence of activities.** To reduce your chance of incurring injury, be sure the cross-training activities you undertake are a service to your marathon goal rather than a drain. For marathon training, which requires building your long run and weekly mileage, it is wise to give up stop-and-go sports (basketball, soccer, etc.) and lateral sports such as tennis until you complete your marathon.

- **Congruence of goals.** Understand that the training necessary to run a fast mile is quite different from that for running a marathon. If you want to include some short-distance races in your marathon training schedule, plan your long run sequences so as not to miss these important workouts.

Make sure your marathon goals are realistic and reflect varying levels of difficulty, with even the most challenging goal attainable for you.

Finding someone to guide and encourage your training can be a great help. If possible, find a coach with a reputation both for enthusiasm and a positive attitude. Such traits can inspire and motivate you. Or join a group whose members share your marathon goals and can provide needed emotional support. It is essential to find fellow runners who run at your approximate pace so that your long runs do not turn into races.

Mental Strategies

Realize that marathon training is not always easy. If running a marathon were simple, there would be no challenge and everyone could do it. To enable you to cope with the physical and mental demands of completing the long training runs and running the actual marathon, particularly when the going gets tough, there are several mental strategies you can adopt. Here are mental preparation tools for meeting the difficulties of the long run.

Self-Talk

Talking to yourself is an easy yet very effective way of keeping yourself on track. Here are phrases you might try saying to yourself:

- "If this were easy, then everybody could complete a marathon."
- "If I quit now, I'll be very disappointed in myself later this afternoon."
- "I'm not really physically tired; I'm more mentally fatigued."
- "In just one more hour this run will be finished, and I'll be at home showering, relaxing, eating."

Imagery and Visualization

Imagine a situation in which you succeed at doing something, and it can become a reality. For example, imagine yourself as a world-class marathoner running in the lead of the Boston Marathon. Imagine that your running form is smooth and graceful. Imagine that you are running effortlessly and very relaxed. You'd be surprised at how much this technique can help you.

Visualization is a vivid way to envision yourself accomplishing your marathon goal. Try these visualizations: Picture yourself running each and every mile of the marathon you are training for. Visualize the finish line with a clock displaying the elapsed time you're shooting for. See in your mind's eye all the spectators cheering for you. Think of all your friends back home pulling for you while you are running.

The Week Before the Marathon

Tapering is a process you'll begin two weeks before a race. You'll notice in the marathon training schedules that week 17 is the taper week. The idea is to slow down. Less is best! Give your body the rest it needs to prepare for the big event. Do not use this time to fit in extra exercise. Your body needs to be loose and rested.

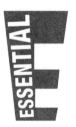

While you're running the race, take time to enjoy the spectators, your fellow runners, and the scenery of the course. Stop negative thoughts dead in their tracks, and change them to positive affirmations. Think about how proud family members and friends will be of you.

Keep stretching as much as possible over the couple of weeks prior to the marathon. Consider getting a leg massage no later than two days before the marathon—although if you've never had a leg massage, don't try it now. Take care of long toenails, blisters, and calluses the week or two prior to the marathon.

As you taper your running, concentrate on reading books and magazine articles that provide you with motivation and inspiration. Take care of any anxieties and mental concerns in the weeks prior to the marathon. Preparation is the best strategy to reduce or eliminate stress and anxiety, which is all the more reason to have completed those key long runs in the weeks prior to the marathon. Similarly, getting a head start on packing if you are traveling out of town for the race is another way to reduce your stress level.

Remember that it is normal to be tense or nervous prior to running a marathon. Even the most seasoned runners experience these feelings. Stay away from participants who are excessively stressed-out or negative so they don't adversely affect your state of mind.

Think about Food

As you scale back the distance and intensity of your running during the last week, realize that you are not burning as many calories. Therefore, you might gain one or two pounds if you don't cut back a bit early in the week on the quantity of your servings. Exercise care in selecting foods to eat during this time period, aiming for nutritionally rich foods rather than simple carbs and high-fat products.

Begin carbohydrate loading three days before the marathon. Choose foods for lunch and dinner that are high in carbohydrates (such as pasta, potatoes, and rice). Don't neglect fruits, vegetables, and some protein sources. Try to really scale back on fats during this time.

Hydrate well the week before the marathon (water is best) and, in particular, during the carbohydrate-loading period three days prior to the marathon. Research shows that carbohydrates convert to glycogen more effectively when consumed with water. If you do gain a couple of pounds, don't worry about it; these fat reserves will serve as fuel during the marathon.

If you are traveling out of town, be sure to pack healthy snack foods to eat the weekend before the marathon. Eliminate the need to search for a grocery store that stocks your favorite foods. If traveling by plane to your marathon destination, check with your airline to see whether you're allowed to carry bottled water with you. If you can't bring your own on board, be sure to let the flight attendant know you'll need several refills while you're in the air. Flying at high altitudes causes dehydration.

Chapter 18

The Marathon Experience

The previous chapter discussed how to train for running the marathon up to the final days. This chapter focuses on the final preparations in the final day or two and on running the marathon itself. This includes racing strategy and injury precautions as well as what to expect and what to do when the marathon is over. Finally, this chapter exposes you to the next level of running—ultra-running.

Physical Preparation

After training so intensely for so long, you're going to feel like you're sabotaging everything by not continuing to work hard the week before the marathon. But listen up: Don't! Stick to your schedule and taper as indicated.

This doesn't mean you should be completely inactive or overeat the week before the race. It's a good idea to stretch as much as possible, always remembering first to warm up your muscles through exercise. In the week prior to the race, take some brisk walks or do some light cycling. Don't do any activity that's going to strain your legs—just something to keep the blood flowing and endorphins up.

On a similar note, if you are traveling to an exciting destination for your marathon and planning on doing some sightseeing by foot, do so no later than two days prior to the race. In fact, if your time is more limited, refrain from taking any long walks the day prior to the marathon. Instead, do your sightseeing from the window of a tour bus or car to conserve your energy for the race.

Packing for an Out-of-Town Marathon

For out-of-town events in particular, don't wait until the night before you travel to collect and pack needed items. Rather, make a list of things you wish to take and begin gathering them in the days prior to departure. Also, pin your race number in advance to the front of your singlet or T-shirt. It's a good idea to take some toilet paper with you to the race site in case there's none remaining when you visit the restrooms.

A day or two before the race, check the weather forecast for the marathon site. Plan and pack for all possible types of weather conditions, given the season. Even if your online weather forecaster predicts great weather for marathon day, conditions can change. Although you can't control the weather, you can prepare for it. Risk overpacking; it's better to have everything you need than to have to buy articles at the last minute in an unfamiliar place.

The Essentials

If you're flying to an out-of-town race, pack your running shoes and essential marathon apparel in carry-on luggage in case your baggage is lost or delayed. Due to variables such as weather conditions and food preference, the following essentials list is suggestive. Try to allow for all contingencies.

- Clothing: singlet*, shorts*, sports bra*, socks*, shoes*, gloves**, hat**, T-shirt (long and short sleeve)**, sweat shirt**, tights**, warm-ups (jacket and long pants)**
- Other handy items: running watch, Vaseline skin lube or Bodyglide, foot powder, handkerchief, shoe laces, small gym bag, lock for locker, towel, race confirmation (to receive race number, if applicable), ibuprofen (or other pain and anti-inflammatory medicine), safety pins, sweat bands, analgesic creams (for example, Ben Gay, Myoflex)
- Possible food items***: Power Bars, gel supplements (for example, GU, Clif Shots, PowerGel), snack items (for example, bagels, whole grain muffins, honey sticks, fruit), carbo-loaded sports drinks, bottled water (*including for the airplane). (Since some airlines no longer allow you to bring bottled liquids on board, check before carrying these onto the plane.)

*If traveling to the race by air, pack these in carry-on luggage.

**Optional items to wear prior to and/or during the marathon. (Consider bringing clothing you can discard during the race after you warm up.)

***Be sure that you have experimented with all food items comprising your pre-race diet.

What About a Cell Phone?

This is a question only you can answer for yourself. Certainly, carrying cell phones everywhere has become part and parcel of the way we live today, so that not having one on you can feel strange. A phone can just as easily clip on your running shorts or leggings as on the waistband of your everyday jeans, or you can carry the phone in a small fanny pack while you run. For long runs and marathons, it's important that the pack you use to carry the phone doesn't chafe or bump against you. Reasons you might want a cell phone on you are:

- **Emergency.** Hey, accidents happen, and despite your careful planning and preparation, bad luck could come your way on race day. If you must stop running for some reason during the marathon, there will be assistance on the course, but having a phone would surely come in handy.
- **Child care.** The time commitment you make to a marathon spans many hours. If you leave children in someone else's care, you may want the caretaker to reach you in an emergency situation.
- **To find someone.** Even if you specify a time and place to meet up with family or friends after the race, circumstances might change. A quick call can save anxious waiting time for everyone involved.

Even with such compelling reasons to have a cell with you, remember that many thousands of people have run and continue to run marathons without cell phones.

Other Travel Considerations

No matter how far you're traveling to the marathon, make sure you arrive in plenty of time. Allow for possible airline or traffic delays so you don't feel rushed. If you're traveling to another time zone, particularly one with a time difference of more than one hour, give yourself time to arrive and acclimate.

The same holds if you'll be running in an environment significantly different from the one you're used to training in. For example, if you live in Maine and you're running a December marathon in Hawaii, try to arrive there at least a week prior to the race to acclimate as much as possible to the higher temperature and humidity you'll experience during the race. Acclimating to heat and humidity takes a minimum of a week. If you've been training in cool or cold temperatures but will be running a marathon in significantly warmer conditions, arriving one to two days prior to the event is not adequate time for your body to acclimate.

Know Where You're Going

Try to find a hotel close to the start and finish of the race. If they're all beyond your budget, already booked, or you want to stay with a friend or family member in the area, map out how you're going to get to the start in plenty of time. Better yet, drive to the race start location the day before to make sure you know the best roads to get there and where you will park. Oftentimes, roads near the course are closed the day of the marathon, thus limiting your access to the start of the race.

Be sure to carefully read all official marathon literature prior to the event to familiarize yourself with procedures (documentation you need to obtain your race number, such as a photo ID, road closures, start and finish line procedures, location of aid stations and portable toilets, and shuttle bus schedules, to name just a few). Don't assume the marathon starting line will be set up adjacent to the site of race headquarters on the day prior (where registration and an exposition is often held), or you will be in for a big shock.

The Final Hours Before the Marathon

The night before and the morning of the race, you're going to be nervous enough that you probably won't want to socialize much, even with your family. You'll want to retire early the night before, taking your mind off the race until the next morning. Ensuring your peace of mind may necessitate spending the money for the convenience of a hotel located near the start of the race. (Plan to stay with friends or family the night following the race, when you'll want to celebrate.)

Be sure to eat proven carbohydrate products during your carbo loading period. Keep pasta sauces simple, avoiding high-fat varieties (for example, alfredo and pesto). Avoid eating salad and vegetables (roughage), which may prove troublesome on race day and cause digestive problems. Stick to water before, during, and after the evening meal. Try to consume at least eight ounces every half-hour. Avoid coffee and tea the night before the race since they may make it difficult for you to fall asleep easily.

Rest and Relax

After your evening meal, try not to think about the marathon any more that evening. Instead, watch television, read (about something other than running), or find something restful to do until turning in for the evening.

Prior to retiring, set two alarm systems to wake you up (alarm clock, wake-up call, running watch alarm setting, cell phone—whatever works). Although this precaution may seem compulsive, the key is to not leave over-sleeping to chance.

Wake up early enough so as not to feel rushed. The few hours before the marathon is a time to relax, yet stay focused as much as possible.

The Pre-Race Morning

Here's a checklist for the morning of your race:

- Wake up early enough to take care of everything you must do (eat and drink, visit the bathroom, dress, and so on).
- If you haven't already done so, formulate a plan to meet your family members or friends at a designated time and place after the race. Have a backup plan if for some reason you are unable to meet at a predetermined time and location after the race.
- Check the weather forecast again for updated information about conditions, temperature range, and wind. Obtaining this information helps in deciding what to wear for most of the marathon. Above all, don't overdress.
- Finally, leave for the race site from your lodging or home with plenty of time to spare, arriving early enough to check any bag and take care of last-minute details. Stay off your feet as much as possible prior to the race. Continue to drink fluids up to 15 minutes before the start of the race. Eat your final snack no later than 30 minutes before the start of the race.

During the Marathon

Runners will start lining up about 15 minutes before the starting time, depending on how big the participant field is. Line up according to your expected pace (faster runners to the front). In a large race, the slower runners can actually create problems (since people tend to be pushed down or slip and fall). Please be courteous!

Also, don't get too caught up in the hoopla by being overly exuberant, yelling and cheering as the gun is about to go off. Save that energy for later when you'll need it. Instead, focus on positive thinking. Visualize all your friends pulling for you and all the hard training you've done for this big race. Take a deep breath, and know that you are not only going to finish the race but achieve your marathon goals.

Pacing

Running at the correct pace for your ability level is crucial in the marathon, especially for the first-time marathoner. It is so easy to start the race running much faster than you have planned or should do. Your pace during the first mile often feels effortless due to your adrenaline rush and the excitement of the event. If you start out too fast, you'll pay dearly for the mistake in the later miles.

A much better strategy is to start out slower than the speed you hope to average and then run the middle miles at your chosen (hopefully realistic) pace. It's a better strategy to pick up the pace during the final miles when you know you can finish rather than starting aggressively. In the world of marathoning, there's no principle of banking the fast miles early in the race and then holding on in the end. If you go that route, you will most assuredly visit the dreaded wall.

Take into consideration weather conditions and course difficulty in predicting your marathon time. Strong winds, high temperatures, driving rains, and hills can add several minutes to your finish time. During the marathon, monitor how you are feeling constantly, and adjust your pace accordingly based on your perceived energy level. Your previous long training runs will provide you with the experience to pace yourself.

Aid Stations

Do not pass up any fluid station. While it's okay to drink water only in the early miles, marathoners must consume sports beverages no later than 60 minutes after beginning to run. Find out through advance practice runs what works best for you.

Water is usually offered at the first tables of an aid station and sports beverages served near the end of the station. If you're not sure whether water or sports drink is in the cup, politely ask. It's not a good feeling splashing what you think is water on your head or chest to cool off and discovering a second or two later that the cool liquid is actually a sports drink!

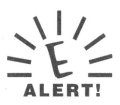

ALERT!

Here's a proven method for drinking while running through the aid stations: Squeeze the top of the cup into a *V* shape to ensure a smooth delivery of fluid directly into your mouth. If you haven't mastered the fine art of drinking on the run (or prefer not to), it's perfectly fine to walk through the aid stations in order to consume the entire contents of the cup.

Supplementing

Many runners are taking advantage of the energy gel products now available to endurance athletes. These provide a fairly quick source of carbohydrate energy. Be sure you chase them down with water to avoid stomach cramps and to ensure absorption.

Some runners stop and eat a power bar, orange slices, jelly beans, etc. to receive needed energy. You don't want to possibly sabotage your race by ingesting something at an unofficial station whose freshness or quality you aren't assured of. Experiment during your long runs with any food products you plan to eat during the marathon, and if they're light enough, think about carrying them in a nonchafing fanny pack. Or consider asking a friend or family member to hand you food at a certain point along the course.

Socializing

Chances are good you will encounter other runners running at your pace during the marathon who engage you in conversation. Whether you wish to stick with them and chat along the way is a personal decision. The positive aspect of socializing is that many great friendships have started this way, and that it can be a good way to take your mind off the physical discomfort you may face later in the marathon. Mutual pacts are often made to provide motivation for each runner to finish.

Another view is that talking might rob you of valuable energy you'll need later. The last miles of the marathon can be quite draining mentally. For that reason alone, you may choose to run the last miles without much conversation. Also, running with someone may slow you down. You'll undoubtedly finish the marathon, but sticking with someone who is slower could compromise your chance of achieving a goal you've set for yourself.

Don't feel you need to be overly sociable at the price of losing sight of your marathon goals. If you really hit it off with someone, ask for her name and then see whether you can track her down through race entry records. A fellow competitor should understand your training investment and accommodate your goal, even if it means being left behind at some point. You certainly don't want to reach the finish knowing in your heart and soul you could have done better. Don't cheat yourself.

On the Course

Once the race is underway, think pacing and overall goals. Remember what you set out to do and monitor yourself so you have the greatest chance to succeed. You will no doubt be buoyed by the energy of the runners around you and of the spectators along the course. Tap into it and let it carry you along, but don't get overzealous and run too fast at first.

Here's where reinforcing self-talk can come in handy, too. Turn your focus inward and remind yourself why you're running. Congratulate yourself for being in the marathon, for realizing your goals, and for being on your way.

For example, a first-time marathoner reminded herself at every mile marker along the way of two different things she was grateful for. Reminding herself of her many blessings became an ongoing way of staying motivated and positive. If you think it might be difficult to come up with fifty-two things (plus a few more when you cross the finish line!), think again—or re-examine your life. Doesn't it feel good to be alive, good to be in an actual race, geared up to run 26.2 miles? Relish the journey.

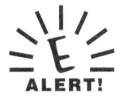
ALERT!

If you feel an increase in pain as you continue to run, seriously consider dropping out of the marathon. No race is worth the risk of causing a minor injury to turn into a major setback.

If you've never run a marathon, there is no way to fully understand in advance the special feelings you will experience during the event. Savor and enjoy each and every moment. Take in all the sites and sounds along the way. High-five the extended hand of a child who views you as an athlete competing at center court. Smile at the spectator telling you, "You're looking strong." Offer some brief words of encouragement to a fellow runner who may not be feeling as strong as you are. Enjoy the diverse scenery along the race course, whether from a bridge you cross, a hill affording a panoramic view of the countryside, or at the sight of storefronts while you cruise down Main Street. Along with the accomplishment of a goal you've worked so hard to achieve, you will be creating memories.

After the Marathon

Right after you finish running, do the following:

- After crossing the line and turning in either the stub on your race number, your index card, or computer chip (each marathon has its own finish line record-keeping system), the first thing you need to do is to get something to drink.
- Determine whether you need to visit the medical tent. Blisters and excessive pain in muscles and joints should be checked out by the medical personnel on hand.

- Within a few minutes of finishing, grab something to eat.
- Stretch thoroughly within 20 minutes of finishing.
- Do not even consider lying down: Keep walking.
- Sign up for a post-race massage (if available).

After you return home or to your hotel, have a nice lunch. This should be a well-balanced meal that includes the majority of calories in carbohydrates. Don't overlook consuming at least 20 percent of total calories from protein sources.

Do not take a nap or lie down for long periods of time (that is, if you don't wish to be very sore or nauseous). Instead, stay on your feet by taking a walk or perhaps going for an easy bike ride of a few miles. Above all, keep moving to minimize leg muscle soreness.

Later that afternoon or evening, go out and celebrate. If you trained properly and followed all of the pre-race and marathon strategies, you should be able to do just about anything you wish (including dancing!). Above all, have a great time.

Post-Marathon Evaluation

The marathon is a mystical event because so many factors come into play in determining how well you do and how much discomfort you will experience. With the marathon behind you, it's now time to think about practices you did correctly along with errors you may have made in your training and racing. Following are evaluation questions to consider in assessing your total marathon experience, both training for and participating in the race. If necessary, modify and adjust your program to address these issues the next time you train for a marathon.

It's important to reflect upon what you might have done better or differently if you had had the chance. If you have any desire to run another marathon (which many runners do), you'll want to make the next one easier and more successful than the one you've just completed.

Marathon Report Card Checklist

You should review your running of the marathon by considering the following: Did you train smart and make it to the starting line healthy and injury free? Did you avoid injury throughout your training, enabling you to complete most of your scheduled workouts? Did you listen to your body and make minor adjustments to your training schedule, thus becoming stronger and not worn down?

Think also about how your training contributed to your marathon performance. Did you train consistently? Did you complete most of the runs (even the 18–23-milers)?

Evaluate your race strategy. Did you eat and drink properly before, during, and after the marathon (and the long training runs)? Did you run at the correct pace for your present ability and conditioning level during the marathon (and the long training runs)? Did you make adjustments for unforeseen problems (for example, blisters, chafing, stomach discomfort, muscle cramps) during the marathon (and the long training runs)?

Finally, think about your mental approach to the marathon. Did you have the best possible psychological attitude during the marathon (and throughout your training)? Were your marathon goals realistic?

Staying Motivated and Combating Burnout

It is not uncommon for runners to experience varying degrees of post-event depression (the blahs, decreased motivation, etc.) after finishing a marathon. This is due in part to achieving a goal that took a lot of time and energy. Now that you have accomplished the goal, you might sometimes feel a void in your life. Until you are ready both mentally and physically to set new goals, consider the following strategies to deal with reduced motivation and/or burnout: Run simply for fun, not worrying about following a training schedule; supplement your running by participating in cross-training activities; take a break from running altogether; spend more time with family and friends, and enjoy more social activities or nonathletic hobbies.

Life After the Marathon

After experiencing the personal satisfaction of completing their first marathon, many runners are interested in returning to their training immediately. Although completing a marathon is quite exciting and therefore motivating, you must take extreme care in the weeks and months following the event to rebuild mileage to pre-marathon levels. The effects on your musculoskeletal system are significant, for your muscles have undergone microtrauma (small tears of the muscle tissue that normally occur as a result of the physical demands of the marathon). These muscular tears require adequate time to heal and regenerate. Jumping right into a heavy training schedule slows down the recovery of muscles and soft connective tissue.

Even if microtrauma damage to your muscles is minimal, your ligaments, joints, and bones are in a vulnerable state immediately following the marathon. To reduce the possibility of an injury, you should take a prudent approach to the full resumption of training.

Some experts argue that runners should take a couple of weeks off with no running after a marathon. However, it is the recommendation of this book that you engage in cross-training activities to maintain cardiovascular fitness, while at the same time allowing your body to heal. Listen to your body and don't push it! If your body tells you that it needs more time to recover, by all means give it the rest that it needs.

Reverse Taper

You should view the next four to six weeks as a reverse taper. No running for the first week will help you recover better than light running would. Do some light runs the second week and build your running back over the subsequent weeks. Eat healthy. A high carbohydrate diet in the first few days after the marathon will help replenish your depleted carbs, and protein will help to rebuild damaged muscle tissue.

With lots of sleep and some easy walks, you'll be ready to run again in no time. Remember that the basic recovery process takes about a month, during which time you should continue to rest, run easy, avoid speed work, and keep your carbohydrate load high. The rule of taking one day of recovery for each mile raced is a rule you should seriously follow. Make sure you take the time to properly recover. If you are having serious pain (more than the usual post-marathon aches and pains), you should plan to visit a sports medicine specialist.

Scheduling Your Next Marathon

Even if you have performed well in one marathon, be careful not to race too soon because you are at a high risk for injury during the next six to eight weeks. Running another marathon, a fast 10K or 10-miler, or deciding to do another 20-mile training run, say, between marathons that are spaced too close together could be enough to cause a lingering injury.

So how long should you wait before running? The answer to that question depends on multiple factors. These include (but are not limited to): your years of running experience; the type and intensity of the training program you've followed with your last marathon; the energy and effort you expended during that marathon; and the duration and completeness of leg recovery after your last marathon.

Most experts say that two marathons are the limit you should run per year (spaced six months apart). The central consideration is that the body needs adequate time to recover from a marathon. Training for and competing in another marathon before your legs have fully recovered can lead to a variety of overuse injuries.

What's Next? Ultra-Running

As if running 26.2 miles weren't quite far enough, ultra-marathoning is becoming increasingly popular. Ultra-marathon events are usually either 50 or 100 miles long. However, there are some events that are more than 100 miles, and there are also 24-hour-long running events.

If after you have run two or three marathons you feel like attempting an ultra-marathon, it is recommended that you do as much research as possible before training for this next step. Research ultra-running and ultra-marathoning Web sites, read running magazines, gather information, and talk to specialists for advice. Whether you work with a coach or an experienced ultra-runner, you should try to find someone who can competently guide you to this next level. To put it mildly, the world of ultra-running is not for everybody. Exercise caution and prudence when attempting something of this magnitude.

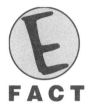

FACT

There are two magazines that are ultra-running's standard bearers. They are *Marathon & Beyond (www.marathonandbeyond.com)* and *Ultrarunning (www.ultraunning.com).* One of the best ultra-marathon Web sites is Kevin Sayers's *www.ultrunr.com.* Another good one is the Extreme Ultrarunning site at *www.extremeultrarunning.com.*

The world of ultra-runners is highly organized through international governing bodies, national organizations, and many clubs. American Ultra-Running Association (AUA) is the United States branch of the International Association of Ultra-Runners (IAU). These organizations develop the rules and policies that most of the popular and legitimate events abide by. The AUA is also a member of the USA Track and Field (USATF). Contact the American Ultra-Running Association (*www.americanultra.org*) to find the club nearest you.

Ultra-Running Events

The events comprising ultra-running vary greatly. The types of races and the way winners are determined are not always the same from race to race. The winners of some of the shorter ultra-marathons, such as the 50-mile races, are determined just like the popular distance races, from the mile race to the marathon: First to cross the finish line wins.

The other type is a fixed-time event. The parameter is given, such as 24 hours, 48 hours, or 6 days. The runner who runs the most miles within that time wins. There are also point-to-point events.

Ultimately, there are no rules in ultra-running. You can stop to eat, rest, walk, and even sleep. It's fairly free and easy. The only penalty is that you are losing time doing these things while your competitors are running.

Training for Ultra-Runs

The training for an ultra-marathon goes way beyond what is described in this book. However, many of the same running principles apply. For example, you cannot jump from here to there. Building mileage slowly and systematically is the key to preparing properly while reducing the likelihood of injury. Stretching is still important.

Physical Preparation

How do ultra-runners cover these long distances, both in training and during the actual events? The evolution of Jeff Galloway's famous walk/run marathon training program can perhaps be traced to the cornerstone of ultra-training, which consists of interspersing running with frequent walking breaks.

The specific ratio of walking to running varies depending largely on the experience and ability level of the ultra-runner. Some throw in a 2-minute walking break for every mile run. Others may find that walking 3 minutes for every 10 minutes running enables them to cover increasingly longer distances.

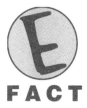

FACT

In the ultra-marathoning world, a series of races known as the Grand Slam is the most renowned. The big four races that comprise the Grand Slam are: Western States 100, Vermont 100, Leadville Trail 100, and Wasatch Front 100. If you complete all of these events in a year, as many ultra-marathoners aspire to do, you would log a total of 400 miles!

For this strategy to be effective, you must implement walking breaks at the beginning of the run or race, not when your leg muscles are at the point of fatigue or breakdown. In short, regularly scheduled walking breaks greatly increase the ultra-runner's range, in comparison with running the entire training or racing distance. Including frequent walking also reduces the wear and tear on the leg muscles, a critical injury prevention strategy.

More competitive ultra-runners integrate advanced training techniques emphasizing strength and endurance into their training schedules. These include speed workouts focusing on longer repeat interval distances (fast-paced running for 800 meters and longer) as well as the inclusion of hill training. In short, their workouts are quite different from that of those racing much shorter distances, such as the 5K or 10K, although they follow the same advanced training guidelines and precautions. However, ultra-runners practice speed work and hill training as discussed in earlier chapters. Nutrition is still paramount. Weight training is still important. And coaches in the sport still caution their runners not to overtrain, if that seems possible in preparing for such an event.

ALERT!

Psychologically, the ultra-marathon requires new adjustments. One of the challenges is finding ways to pass hours and hours of time mentally. Ultra-runners comment that there is no limit to the variety of topics they think about while running, ranging from the practical and conventional to the absurd!

Other Preparations

Nutritionally, ultra-marathoners eat greater quantities, and they eat more frequently during their events than marathoners. Their training schedules tend to be made up of more long runs than in those of marathoners. Because the weather conditions during these extra-long events can change drastically (due to topographical variations of the course along with the range from morning to night), ultra-runners must be prepared to add or strip multiple layers of clothing at a moment's notice. The same changeability can be said about terrain. One minute these athletes are running through the desert, and an hour later they may be climbing a mountain. An ultra-runner has to be thoroughly prepared for competing in such an event.

Chapter 19

Girls (Women!) Just Want to Have Fun

Everyone knows the adage that men and women are different. In the world of running, women and men differ, as well—though both sexes have achieved incredible results. Are the differences profound or significant enough for women to have an entire section of this book dedicated to them? The answer is a resounding, "Yes!"

Comparing Men and Women Runners

Before detailing significant differences, it's important to point out that there are many similarities between men and women runners. First, the biomechanics of running does not differ between men and women. Posture and stride affect male and female runners in the same way. Neither do training techniques vary from men to women. Both men and women can and should follow the various training schedules provided in this book. With little or no variation, both men and women can do the speed workouts, cross-training, weight-training, and stretching discussed in previous chapters. Additionally, men and women routinely run in the same races.

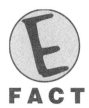

FACT

Amazingly, it wasn't until 1900 that women's events were included in the Olympic games, and it wasn't until 1928 that women's track and field was added. In that year, American Betty Robinson won a gold medal in the 100-meter race.

In any of these areas, little separates the two sexes. However, there are also numerous factors that are specific to the female runner. Let's cover a few of the differences here.

Body Type

Women runners do tend to carry more body fat than men—approximately 5–10 percent more. Body fat is dead weight, and women need to exert more energy to carry that weight, which saps their strength and stamina. Men tend to have larger hearts and lungs, which deliver oxygenated blood faster and in greater quantity than those of their female counterparts. This allows muscles to respond better and faster. Men also tend to have greater muscle mass and stronger bones.

This is not to say that there aren't women runners who finish ahead of men in a lot of races. However, these biological differences explain why elite male runners are almost always faster than accomplished women of track and field. This is particularly true in sprinting. However, the gap in performance between elite-caliber men and women narrows as race distances become longer. This is especially so in race distances of the marathon and longer.

Menstruation

Just because the discomforts of monthly menstruation are commonplace for women doesn't mean they go unnoticed. Menstrual side effects (bloating, cramps, mood swings) can affect women's very participation and performance in both training and racing. At certain times, heavy menstrual flow and/or severe cramps may keep some women from exercising at all.

Although the prospect of strapping on a pair of running shoes and shorts and hitting the pavement may not seem appealing to women during menstruation, it's important to remember that exercise at such a time is an excellent activity. The very act of sweating is an effective antidote to menstrual bloating, which is a form of water retention.

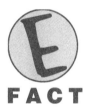

FACT

Menstruation need not interfere with your competitive urges. Many women runners report little to no change in racing results when they run competitively during their menstrual period. Even when they run with mental and/or physical discomfort, running seems to make women feel better in the end.

Many women runners who exercise regularly find they suffer less-severe cramps and are less affected by menstrual side effects than are women who do not exercise. The other side is that there are women who no longer menstruate regularly or at all because they overdo exercise in both training and racing. Even though this might not seem like such a bad thing, infrequent or irregular menstrual cycles, called *amenorrhea,* can lead to an early onset of osteoporosis and interfere with childbearing. It is strongly recommended that women runners discuss their running habits and their monthly menstrual cycle with their doctor from time to time to make sure they are neither overdoing exercise nor neglecting important health concerns.

Fitness for Prenatal Women

Exercise plays an important part in a healthy pregnancy. Assuming there are no complications, a woman should try to exercise throughout the duration of pregnancy. Some studies suggest that full benefits are not realized if women stop exercising partway through pregnancy. Of course, if your doctor recommends that you stop exercising due to concerns about your health or the health of the fetus, then by all means stop.

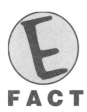

FACT

According to the American College of Obstetricians and Gynecologists (ACOG), "Regular exercise improves a pregnant woman's physical and mental health. Exercising and being fit help a woman during pregnancy and may improve her ability to cope with the pain of labor. Exercise will also make it easier for a woman to get back in shape after the baby is born."

Running Versus Walking

It is important to discuss with your doctor your jogging, running, and/or walking while pregnant. The ability to run well into the second trimester is a decision you must make with your doctor, since women's bodies respond differently to the same athletic stresses. Many doctors, while not insisting you give up exercise, might warn you either to reduce the intensity of running or stop altogether, substituting walking. It is very important that you and your doctor make this decision together. Many women are loath to give up running until their additional weight slows them down. Don't press yourself in this situation. Walking is an excellent substitute.

Now that more prenatal (before the birth) and postnatal (after the birth) women are exercising, learning about the effects of exercise continues apace. In 2003, the ACOG revised its guidelines on exercise during pregnancy and postpartum. ACOG's previous recommendation for pregnant women to exercise at a limited heart rate has been revised to emphasize that women exercise at a moderate and comfortable level. (Read ACOG's guidelines for exercise during pregnancy at *www.acog.org/publications/ patient_education/bp119.cfm.*)

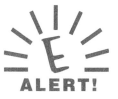

ALERT!

For some women, exercise during pregnancy is not recommended. If your doctor gives you the go-ahead to start a fitness program, you should monitor yourself during exercise for any warning signs of a problem. If any health issues surface, immediately contact your doctor for further guidance.

Taking a Prenatal Exercise Class

Some women find that taking part in a supervised exercise class provides assurance and support. Before enrolling in any prenatal program, find out whether the program meets the following criteria:

- The instructor has a fitness or health-related degree and experience or training in obstetrics.
- The instructor is competent to answer fitness- and pregnancy-related questions.
- The instructor incorporates ACOG guidelines and knows warning signs and symptoms regarding pregnancy.
- You are required to provide a health history and physician's consent before joining the class.
- There is an established procedure for management of injuries or emergencies.
- The facility is appropriate for prenatal exercise, having a supportive floor, mats, nearby restrooms, and exercise room kept cool.
- The safety and comfort of the participants are never sacrificed.
- The class accommodates varying levels of fitness.

- The class provides frequent breaks to check level of exertion and to hydrate.
- The class includes a warm-up, aerobic exercise, strength and flexibility exercises, and a cool-down.
- The class includes pregnancy-specific exercises such as for lower back flexibility and pelvis.

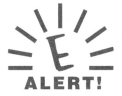

ALERT!

Catherine Cram, an exercise physiologist who specializes in prenatal and postnatal fitness, offers the following advice for a safe and effective prenatal exercise program: "Reassess your fitness goals, listen to your body, and consider a supervised prenatal exercise class with a qualified instructor."

Shoes and Clothing

Wear shoes during pregnancy that are one-half to one size larger to allow room for foot swelling. Shoes with Velcro closures make frequent adjustments easier. Clothing should be comfortable. If overheating is a problem, wear nonconstricting clothing that breathes and wicks moisture away from the body to help it stay cool. A sports bra with wide shoulder straps can provide good support, help protect the breasts, and ease or prevent shoulder discomfort.

Forget about Calories

A woman should never exercise to lose weight while pregnant and should not attempt to prevent weight gain through restricted calories. Mother and fetus need an extra 300 calories a day (for multiple-birth pregnancies, add 300 calories per fetus). To determine whether you are eating enough, you should monitor your body weight regularly.

Pregnant women can expect to gain 25–35 pounds. Lean, athletic women who have low levels of body fat before pregnancy may need to gain more. Women who fall into this latter category can take comfort in knowing that they will recover quickly. If you are pregnant but are not gaining weight (or are losing weight), you need to increase your caloric intake of nutrient-rich foods. Pregnancy may not be an athletic event, but it is physically very demanding. It is important to remember that the new life developing in the womb needs nutrients and calories to grow and be healthy.

Fitness for Postnatal Women

During the postnatal period, a woman's body works hard to return to its condition prior to pregnancy. This process can take nearly as long as the pregnancy itself, so be patient. Muscle and skin that stretched to allow for your baby's growth take time to regain their original tone and can make fitting into your old wardrobe challenging. Although this can be emotionally discouraging, it is normal.

The following are prenatal and postnatal fitness guidelines:

- **Frequency:** Exercise 3–5 times per week.
- **Intensity:** Exercise at a level that feels somewhat hard to hard.
- **Time:** Those just starting an exercise program should do an aerobic activity for only 5–10 minutes at a time. Those who were fit prior to pregnancy can exercise for 20–45 minutes.

Get Your Doctor's Approval

As in the prenatal stage, a woman in the postnatal period should get approval from her doctor or health care provider before engaging in exercise. If approval is given, follow postnatal fitness guidelines until the postnatal period is over (after six to twelve months).

The new mother's postnatal condition affects the start of exercise as well as the type. In addition to postnatal physiological adjustments, one of the biggest fitness challenges to a new mother consists in finding available free time to workout. With a little planning, however, a new mother can carve out a piece of her busy day for exercise that enhances her physical and emotional health.

Finding Time to Exercise

New parents can designate certain times of the day (or evening) when each of them takes care of the baby exclusively. This arrangement allows each spouse to have some personal time for exercise.

A rotational schedule in which extended family members or friends take care of your baby enables you as a new mother to have time to exercise. Schedule this time as you would a class or an appointment. Designating a start and a finish exercise time will help you to recruit caretakers and communicates your respect for their time.

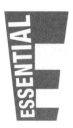

Exercise for new mothers is at least as important as going out for the evening. Make an appointment with yourself and arrange a babysitter at regular times. Unless you are training for a marathon, as little as an hour of exercise time can make a huge difference in your fitness level.

Baby-Friendly Equipment

Today's baby-friendly equipment makes it possible for baby to safely go along on Mom and Dad's walks, jogs, runs, and bike rides. The baby jogger-runner is more stable and durable than a conventional stroller. For bicycling, there are numerous options for baby and child apparatus, such as screened-in trailers, child seats, and mounted tandem attachments. For safety's sake, be sure that both you and your child wear helmets.

Osteoporosis and Menopause

Osteoporosis, a disease of brittle bones that affects a great many women, can mean the unfortunate end to your running career. The jarring action of running or a quick fall can cause a fracture. When bone mass begins to decline around the age of thirty-five, women become vulnerable to osteoporosis. The process, if undetected, can accelerate after menopause. However, young women with diets low in iron and calcium who place too much stress on their bodies can also contract this disease.

Osteoporosis cannot be reversed. If an affected woman detects osteoporosis early enough, she can slow the disease's progress with the help of her doctor. A calcium-rich diet is a primary way of retarding osteoporosis, as is running. Even though running places stress on bones, it at the same time acts as an agent to build stronger bones by automatically increasing bone density in areas of greatest stress. If you are a woman runner, you should discuss osteoporosis with your doctor at your next medical appointment.

Menopause

Menopause is a difficult time for some women, less so for others. Although it can involve deep mood swings, hot flashes, and other discomforts, it need not discourage women from running. There has been no conclusive evidence that running (or other kinds of exercise) increases or decreases the main effects of menopause. However, there is little doubt that exercise is a wonderful antidote to stress, depression, anxiety, and a host of other less desirable emotions.

Since menopause can take as long as ten years to complete its cycle, many aging women lose their desire and motivation to continue running. Regardless, countless dedicated women have continued running right through their entire menopause, never losing the enjoyment and richness that running brings to their lives. Again, consulting with your physician is your best way to run through menopause without physical or mental discomfort.

Safety Tips for Women Runners

Though people like to think they live in an enlightened time when women are safe running by themselves, it's always a good idea to be aware of potentially unpleasant or dangerous situations. Here are commonsense suggestions to keep you safe.

- Don't run in isolated areas, particularly after dark.
- Whenever possible, run with other people after dark.

- Vary your running routine. Don't run in the same place at the same time on the same day.
- Mix up your schedule so strangers can't anticipate when and where you run.
- Tell a family member, roommate, or friend of your route and approximately what time you expect to return.
- Bring a whistle, panic button device, or some other way to attract attention should a threat materialize.
- If possible, learn self-defense tactics.

The "Cult" of Female Runners

Ask women what they enjoy about running and though their answers will vary, you will find common themes. These include escape, camaraderie, energy, staying in shape, and personal success. While women have more opportunities than ever, they also carry more responsibilities as they juggle home, career, relationships, child-rearing, and so on. Maintaining the balancing act is hard enough; often it causes a rupture in the form of divorce, injury, or empty-nest syndrome. Running—whether alone or in groups—is a gift women give themselves, allowing a healing place where no one who isn't invited usually intrudes. As Jennifer Lin and Susan Warner reflect in an article in *Training Zone Sports*, "We run to escape, to relax, to hammer out life's problems to the beat of rubber soles on pavement. It is our therapy, our time to mull questions big and small."

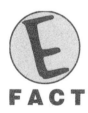

FACT

In 2008, the Susan G. Komen Race for the Cure will celebrate its 25th anniversary. The Race for the Cure is a 5K event that raises money for breast cancer research and awareness. Since 2005 alone, over one million runners have participated in the Race for the Cure, which is now staged in nearly every state in the United States as well as in several international locations. For more information, go to *www.komen.org*.

Women-Only Races

As the number of women runners grows, it is easier to find races for women only. Sponsors are aware that women love to run together, especially to support worthy causes. Any woman who has run in a woman-only race knows there is something especially bonding about the experience. In 2005, the ten women's races with the largest number of finishers hosted over 40,000 runners—and that's just the top ten races! They were:

1. The Revlon Run for Women 5K in Los Angeles, California (the fourth largest race in the United States in 2005)
2. The St. Luke's Women's Fitness Celebration 5K in Boise, Idaho
3. The Tufts Health Plan for Women 10K in Boston, Massachusetts
4. The Race for the Cure and Quad Cities 5K in Rock Island, Illinois
5. The Circle of Friends Mini 10K in New York, New York
6. The Freihofer's Run for Women 5K in Albany, New York
7. The Women's 5K Classic in Allentown, Pennsylvania
8. The Race for the Cure 5K in San Francisco, California
9. The Montana Woman's Run 2 Mile in Billings, Montana
10. The More Half-Marathon in New York, New York

Chapter 20

Running Away from Home

Running is a sport you can take with you wherever you go. Remember, the great thing about running is that you really only need your shorts, shirt, and shoes to make it happen. So when you're planning a trip for business or pleasure, don't forget to pack your running gear.

20

Packing Your Running Gear

Here's how to pack your gear: Designate two small bags for your running gear. One is for your running shoes (a plastic shopping bag is good for these) and the other for your running clothes and necessary accessories. In this second bag put either your warm-weather gear (shorts, short-sleeve T-shirt or singlet, running bra, etc.) or your cold-weather gear (leggings, thermal top, running bra, long-sleeve T-shirt, gloves, hat, etc) as well as your all-important running watch for all seasons. Even if you're going someplace cold and need extra gear, this won't weigh much. Wouldn't you rather lug around the extra pounds your gear weighs than the extra pounds you'll weigh if you don't run while you're gone?

But It's a Vacation!

True, vacations are times when you leave the stresses and worries of your daily routine behind and indulge in the good life. For many people that means rest, relaxation, and fun like sightseeing, dining out, dancing, sunbathing, and other leisure activities. Do you see running on this list? No. Would most of your friends call you crazy if you told them you were looking forward to running your 5 miles a day on your trip to the Grand Canyon? Probably, but remember: It's your time off, not theirs!

Reasons to Run on Vacation

Think of it this way: If you have set up a running routine to get in shape and lose weight, you're probably already seeing results and enjoying running by now. When you go on vacation and indulge in big meals, drinking, and extra sleep, those pounds and inches will come back in no time—unless, of course, you can get in a few runs. Even short runs will keep your metabolism humming and ensure you don't regress. You'll enjoy that piña colada even more knowing you've earned it through aerobic exercise.

If you're in training for a half-marathon or marathon, or not, getting miles in for a couple of weeks could throw you off. You don't want to undermine all the hard work and training miles you've put in by not keeping up with your running during the trip.

"I Was Going to Run But..."

Many runners have given any number of reasons for not performing their workouts when out of town. Although it's great to have fun and break away from your normal routine when traveling, it's important not to let your running go on vacation, particularly if you're training for an event just a few short weeks away. Feelings of worry and guilt can arise upon viewing those blank spaces in your training log. If only you had done things differently!

Planning ahead greatly increases the likelihood that you will maintain your training while away. Long before your departure, your first step is to research all your options concerning when and where you can run.

Oftentimes, running first thing in the morning proves the best solution, particularly when your agenda is quite full. But it's also important to be realistic. If you expect to be partying well past midnight at a wedding reception, will you have the self-discipline and motivation to follow through with your plan to run early the next morning?

If you're traveling with family members, it's important to consider their needs. Are there activities they can do while you're out running? Who will be watching the kids for the hour or so that you're away? How will you work it out so that your partner also has some private time?

Lodging Considerations

Where you decide to stay can also affect the likelihood you will run when out of town. Hotels that have fitness centers equipped with treadmills make running easy. Some accommodating hotels in big cities have mapped out running routes of various distances that begin and end at their front door. If your hotel doesn't have workout facilities on-site, ask management whether they have special arrangements with a nearby gym that their guests can use at reduced rates or even for free.

If you prefer staying at an economy motel when away, select one located adjacent to residential neighborhoods or on a road with sidewalks and light traffic so that it will be both safe and convenient to run directly from your room. You can always hop in your car to run in another part of town if you don't feel comfortable with your motel's location.

If you will be staying at the home of friends or relatives, let them know in advance that you plan to run so they will be supportive of your training. They might be able to suggest a good running route nearby or have runner friends who would welcome you to join them.

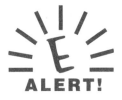

ALERT!

If there is absolutely no way to fit in a workout during your weekend getaway, modify your training schedule to fit in those important runs before leaving. Be sure not to cluster too many days of running back-to-back, though, since doing so can lead to injury.

If you're going away to rekindle the romance in your relationship and your significant other is not a runner, remind him or her (and yourself) that regular exercise helps you feel and look better. It improves your circulation, overall health, energy level, mental acuity, and appetite—all important for a healthy sex life! In fact, perhaps the two of you can begin participating in exercise together while away. It's an ideal way to bond and have fun.

Run to See the Sights

Besides the very important and real benefits of maintaining your fitness regimen while you're on the road, the greatest satisfaction in running away from home is in exploring new places, runners often proclaim. Let's face it, there's nothing like running through a new neighborhood to reinvigorate your runs. It's fun to see how people in other parts of the country (and the world) decorate their homes and yards, configure their streets, and go about their daily lives. Not only are you getting your exercise in, but you're getting an up-close-and-personal look at a new part of the world. You'll be amazed at how invigorating this is.

Don't be surprised if you start remembering your trips by the runs you took instead of the meals you ate, the museums you visited, even the family stories you heard for the first time. When you're on your run, the time is yours. Even if only a quick 20 minutes, running on your own in a new place revives all your senses.

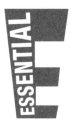

If you've gotten into the good habit of keeping a running log or journal, this will come in handy when you're traveling. Take notes about what you have liked best about your run and what you have liked least. In this way, your running log becomes your travel journal.

Planning for Safety

If adventure is one side of the equation in running while away from home, safety is the other. Because as exciting as it is to be in new places, the truth is that you're not in familiar territory. Taking a wrong turn on foot somewhere can get you lost more easily than you think. If you don't speak the native language, have no map with you, or find yourself in the dark, you could be in big trouble. And though most runners agree that it's particularly gratifying to do some of these runs alone, running by yourself exposes you to more dangers—anything from twisting your ankle while running on a trail to accidentally running into the bad part of town.

Use Common Sense

Such frightening scenarios are easily avoided by following common-sense safety rules. First, trust your instincts. If a business trip on a limited budget puts you in a hotel where there's nothing but strip malls and highways everywhere you look, you may have to either use the hotel gym or limit your run to laps around the parking lot. You certainly don't want to be running anywhere near a busy street or highway where cars are making quick turns or going at high speeds, not to mention feeling vulnerable in a setting like this.

Likewise, if you're a bit behind schedule and you get to your hotel, campsite, or bed and breakfast at dusk instead of earlier in the afternoon, however beautiful the setting, you should consider postponing your run until morning when you have the full advantage of daylight. Once you know a trail or an area and have gauged how far it is to run, then you may want to consider running at dusk. But don't run anywhere new in the dark.

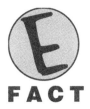

FACT

There are certain areas in life where risk-taking can pay off big time. Running on the road is not one of them. If you wouldn't want a member of your family or one of your best friends to go out on the run you're considering, then don't do it yourself.

Another commonsense safety rule is to leave a message with someone that you're going for a run. If you're traveling by yourself, you should leave a note in your hotel room, tent, or wherever you're staying. Indicate the time you are leaving and how long you expect to be out.

Another easy and practical thing to do is ask at the front desk whether there's a running trail accessible from the hotel. The staff is usually happy to tell you all about it, including whether there are loops of different lengths in case you want to do 3 miles one day and 10 another, for example. After getting the lowdown from the staff, you can let them know that you're going out on that trail and you expect the run to take you, say, a half-hour. Leave your name and your room number with the hotel personnel.

If you're traveling with others, make sure they know to expect you back within a certain time. Be generous with your estimate of the time but not overly so. You don't want them calling the police if you're not back in 45 minutes like you said because you decided to run a bit farther. On the other hand, you don't want them to figure you're just out enjoying yourself if you're not back within a few hours.

While on your run, carry identification with you. Write your name, home address, and phone number and the name, address, and phone number of the place where you're staying on a piece of paper that you can tuck into a pocket or gear holder. Don't wear anything that could make you a target, such as sparkling jewelry or your most expensive wristwatch.

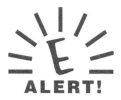

ALERT!

When running in a new place, you need a fanny pack or a wrist or ankle attachment that can hold a few small things like your hotel key, a few dollars in pocket change, and certainly identification. You'll need to feel comfortable but not conspicuous.

You must wear or carry a timepiece with you. Best, of course, is your waterproof, lightweight stopwatch or training watch that you've bought along with your other necessary gear for running. But if you have forgotten it, wear or carry your regular watch. Since you'll be setting off into the unknown, time is your best bearing.

Plan to run 15–20 minutes out, then 15–20 minutes back. Because your senses are working overtime to take in everything new, running toward your destination will seem to take longer than your return trip. Keep an eye on your watch. You'll feel like you've been running for longer than your watch says, but when you get to the halfway point and start to head back, you'll enjoy reliving sights from the run out, and time will go by more quickly.

More Safety Tips

There's an excellent Web site called Run the Planet (*www.runtheplanet .com*) that's loaded with advice on where and when to run throughout the world. Here are especially good tips from a section called "Stay Safe While Running" by the Hudson Mohawk Road Runners Club:

- Take a whistle with you.
- Know where police are usually to be found and where businesses, stores, and offices are likely to be open and active.
- Do not wear a radio/headset/earphones or anything that distracts you so that you are completely unaware of your environment.
- Take notice of who is ahead of you and who is behind you. Know where the nearest public sites are with some general activity—there is usually safety in numbers.

- When in doubt, follow your intuition and avoid potential trouble. If something seems suspicious, do not panic but run in a different direction.
- If the same car cruises past you more than once, take down even a partial license number and make it obvious that you are aware of its presence (but keep your distance).
- Do not approach a car to give directions or the time of day. Point toward the nearest police or information source, shrug your shoulders, but keep moving. If you feel you must respond, do it while moving.
- Do not panic. Do not run toward a more isolated area.
- Use discretion in acknowledging strangers. Be friendly, but keep your distance and keep moving.

Running with Others

Depending on the type of travel you're doing, it may be easy for you to join up with other runners—or not. If you're on a business trip with associates whom you know also run, you can ask them whether they want to meet for a group run. If you're at a large hotel or convention center, ask the staff of the health club whether they know of any guests at the hotel who might want to run with someone. Or you might see another runner in the lobby when you come down for your run, in which case think about going together.

Just don't shed common sense in your enthusiasm to explore and exercise. If the hotel hooks you up with someone who doesn't seem like your type, make up an excuse to get out of the run. It's your personal time, and you are not obligated to run with someone even if the hotel did the work to find a running partner for you. Likewise, don't be offended if this other person seems to lose interest in running with you. No big deal—just go enjoy your run.

Running with Business Associates

Remember, too, that if you're on a business trip, you might end up jogging alongside the CEO—or a new assistant. In the same way that it's unprofessional to drink too much at a company function and start gossiping, the same holds true for informal meetings like runs. If the CEO wants your opinion about the department you work in, find something positive to say (even if you're miserable), at least to start the conversation. If he prods you, be tactful. You want to leave a senior manager with the impression that you're a team player and a smart person, someone who understands where the company is going and has constructive ideas about how to contribute.

If you don't have ideas, here's your opportunity to see whether the CEO will share his vision with you. Ask what his favorite aspects of the job are or how his prior experience is influencing his current position. Most people love to talk about themselves.

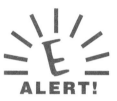

ALERT!

When you're sharing in a positive activity like running, it's easy to feel an instant camaraderie with someone. In a business setting, however, don't mistake this for a window to tell all. You don't have to talk about business at all if you don't want to. Instead, talk about where you run at home, races you've run, or how long you've been running.

Racing on the Road

A way to get an invigorating workout while on a business or pleasure trip is to enter a local race. Go online a few weeks before you're scheduled to leave and do a search for local running clubs in the area you're planning to visit. Go to their Web sites, and see what's on the race calendar. Call the contact person for the race to get more information on the size of the event, whether it's a hilly or flat course, whether there's a post-race party or fair, and so on. If you decide to do the race, ask for directions from the place where you'll be staying and ask how long it should take to get there.

Marathoning Around the World

Why not do a really big race in a new place? That's what legions of marathoners from around the world choose to do. The many advantages are that you can get a good rate to travel and stay someplace for a week, you're traveling with like-minded folks, you don't have to worry too much about how much you eat while you're there (though, of course, you want to avoid foods that are too exotic, especially before the race), and you'll have an instant sightseeing tour.

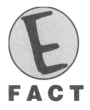

FACT

Many cities have special races to celebrate holidays like Thanksgiving, Halloween, Memorial Day, Labor Day, and New Year's. New York City's Midnight Run on New Year's Eve draws thousands of runners from all over the world to run a 5K through Central Park at midnight, accompanied by fireworks and nonalcoholic champagne. It's an extremely festive and fun way to start a new year.

It's easy to find information on running marathons in all corners of the world. Start at *www.runnersworld.com*, or buy *Runner's World* magazine, and you'll be on your way.

Favorite Running Cities

The folks at *Runner's World* decided to rate the twenty-five best cities for running in the United States. How did they do it? According to them, they "tabulated the number of running clubs and races in the largest U.S. cities….how much park area is available in each city for runners, how average precipitation levels and temps compared to the competition, and even how crime rates stacked up…." Their system is quite impressive and is detailed on their Web site at *www.runnersworld.com* under "The 25 Best Running Cities." Their annotated list provides runners with a "must run," a favorite race, a celebrated place to eat, and where to get help in that city. Here's their list of the Top 25:

1. San Francisco, California
2. San Diego, California
3. New York City, New York

4. Chicago, Illinois
5. Washington, D.C.
6. Minneapolis/St. Paul, Minnesota
7. Boulder, Colorado
8. Boston, Massachusetts
9. Denver, Colorado
10. Portland, Oregon
11. Austin, Texas
12. Seattle, Washington
13. Philadelphia, Pennsylvania
14. Colorado Springs, Colorado
15. Dallas, Texas
16. Anchorage, Alaska
17. Raleigh, North Carolina
18. Salt Lake City, Utah
19. Honolulu, Hawaii
20. Atlanta, Georgia
21. Houston, Texas
22. Phoenix, Arizona
23. Madison, Wisconsin
24. Monterey, California
25. Fort Collins, Colorado

Some Personal Favorites

The following list describes the top running cities in the United States that this runner finds particularly special.

New York, New York

Nothing beats running in Central Park, an oasis in one of the biggest and most exciting cities in the world. Strap on your running shoes and prepare to be wowed. You'll join thousands of runners on their daily loops through Central Park, become one with fellow exercisers on Rollerblades and bicycles, pass horse-drawn carriages, and see strollers of every nationality. You'll pass the famous restaurant Tavern on the Green and where the New York City Marathon concludes as well as the monumental and lovely Metropolitan Museum of Art.

Head uptown to the Reservoir, where joggers have a 1.5-mile trail practically all to themselves with some of the best views of the skyline you can find. The New York City Road Runners Club sponsors races almost every weekend, including fun ones with various themes. There's no better way to feel connected to this imposing city as a traveler than to participate in the ritual of running with the natives.

Chicago, Illinois

From wherever you're staying in Chicago, it's not far to Lake Shore Drive, which runs along the shores of Lake Michigan. Yes, this is a roadway, but there's a walking and running path that parallels it. Talk about some nice skyline views! You'll get a great perspective on the Windy City as you run past Soldier Field, the aquarium, the art museum, the pier, and down to the more residential part of town. Depending on the time of year, be prepared for weather conditions ranging from humidity to arctic air. One thing's for sure: That breeze off the lake will either aid or challenge you. What better way to gear up for a night of blues music and barbecue than to get in a run before dinner?

Waterbury, Vermont

With the world-class ski resorts of Stowe and Sugarbush close by, Waterbury is an almost picture-perfect Vermont town of church spires, antique shops, and quaint village streets. And then there are the foothills of the Green Mountains. You can't run in Waterbury without going up them—and down them. But your legs won't mind when your senses are filled with the beauty of Vermont on a fall day, or blanketed in new snow, or turning green in spring. Even summer provides a visual feast of mottled sun and shade ripe with the scent of pine. If you're not used to running hills, though, take it easy going up and down. An old saying says that going down is for your legs; going up is for your heart. Enjoy the challenge.

Washington, D.C.

One of the country's most popular marathons is the Marine Corps Marathon, called both "the People's Marathon" and "the Monuments' Marathon." Why? Because the 26.2-mile course snakes through the monuments of our nation's capital, including the Capitol, the Pentagon, the Smithsonian Institution, the Kennedy Center, and the Lincoln, Jefferson, and Washington Monuments. It's a race and a history lesson all in one. As a business or leisure traveler, you don't have to run the whole marathon course to experience the beauty and history in and around this city. And the areas adjacent to downtown Washington, such as Georgetown and Arlington, Virginia, are also beautiful for running and touring.

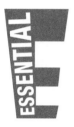

Whether your travels take you to one of these top-rated running cities or not, you're guaranteed great memories if you follow the advice in this chapter and run away from home. It's addicting!

Charleston, South Carolina

Charleston was first settled in 1670, ranking it one of this country's oldest and most historic cities. The area is quite diverse culturally, recreationally, and geographically, with much to see and do. Charleston's charm and beauty is characterized by beautiful beaches, parks, antebellum plantations, tidal creeks and marshes, and a lovely downtown historic district.

Without question, the best way to tour Charleston is not by one of its famous carriage tours but rather by foot. Stay downtown or park at Colonial Lake, the City Marina, the Battery, Waterfront Park, or the South Carolina Aquarium to begin your run or walk. The pedestrian sidewalks on several of Charleston's bridges offer spectacular views of the Charleston peninsula, harbor, Ashley and Cooper Rivers, marshes, and more. Two of these include the James Island Connector and the Arthur Ravenel Jr. Bridge. The latter is also the central attraction for the 40,000-plus participants who run or walk the Cooper River Bridge Run 10K, held in early spring.

Other recreational sites that offer paths on which to take in beautiful sights include Hampton Park as well as James Island, Palmetto Islands, and Wannamaker County Parks. Drive to any of the three barrier islands (Folly Beach, Sullivan's Islands, and Isle of Palms) and run on the beach or through the neighborhoods in these beautiful communities.

Finding a Running Club, at Home or Abroad

A Couple of Clicks Away

There are a number of excellent running clubs around the world that are easy to find, inexpensive to join, and that sponsor activities you can participate in on either a particular weekend or all year. Belonging to a running club is a good way to stay motivated, learn from others, meet people with similar interests, and participate in challenging events. Some clubs are big—like those associated with well-known marathons such as the Boston Athletic Club and the New York Road Runners' Club. Sparsely populated areas have smaller clubs. Different clubs have different personalities.

Search via Yahoo! and Google for "running club + [the name of your town, state initials]" (for example, "running club + Kimberton, PA"). You're bound to find a lot of interesting sites, even if they aren't what you were originally looking for.

Clubs in the United States

In the United States, the best place to start is with the granddaddy of them all, the Road Runners' Club of America (RRCA) at *www.rrca.org*. Not only can you find local and national club listings through the RRCA, you can get an idea of what's happening with running across the country. To find clubs in the state where you live or a state you're planning to visit, you can go straight to a map on their Web site, click on the state, and immediately access a list of all the running clubs in that state. The RRCA's full contact information is as follows:

RRCA National Office

1501 Lee Highway, Suite 140
Alexandria, VA 22209
Phone: (703) 525-3890
✑ *www.rrca.org*

Clubs in Canada

Like the United Sates, Canada has lots of running clubs that offer organized events for their members and guests. One of the top sites to search for clubs in Canada and in other countries (as well as in the United States) is The Running Network. They're at:

Running Network, LLC

28 W. Milwaukee St.
P.O. Box 801
Fort Atkinson, WI 53538-0801
Phone: (608) 827-0806
✑ *www.runningnetwork.com*

Outside of the United States and Canada

Run the Planet at *www.runtheplanet.com* provides an excellent international directory. If you search on the site for running clubs, you'll be directed to pages of national and international listings. Besides the United States and Canada, you can look up clubs in Africa, Antarctica, Asia, Europe, Oceania, and South America. In the "Race Calendar" section, you'll find information on races in Austria, Belgium, Switzerland, Serbia and Montenegro, the Czech Republic, Germany, Denmark, Spain, Finland, France, the United Kingdom, Greenland, Greece, Hungary, Ireland, Iceland, Italy, Luxembourg, Latvia, the Netherlands, Norway, Poland, Portugal, Romania, Russia, Sweden, and Slovenia. What's to stop you? Run the Planet is also a treasure trove of information about all aspects of running, including its history.

Appendix B

Magazines and Books
on Running

Magazines

With the explosion of information available on the Internet, you'd think magazines and books would be obsolete. However, the ever-expanding selection of magazines, periodicals, and books is a testament to the fact that nothing quite beats the tactile experience of hands-on reading.

Sure you can find out all kinds of information online, even race calendars, but there's nothing like finding it all in one place in your running magazine. Some of the most popular and well-known running magazines are listed below. Check 'em out!

Runner's World—**"the worldwide authority on running information"**

Rodale, Inc.
Emmaus, PA 18099
Phone: (610) 967-8809
✑ *www.runnersworld.com*

Running Journal—**"the source for road racing and fitness news in the Southeast"**

P.O. Box 157
Greeneville, TN 37744
Phone: (423) 638-4177
✑ *www.running.net*

Running Research News—**"a monthly newsletter which keeps sports-active people up-to-date on the latest information about training, sports nutrition, and sports medicine."**

P.O. Box 27041
Lansing, MI 48909
Phone: (517) 371-4897
✑ *www.rrnews.com*

Running Times—**"the runner's best resource"**

213 Danbury Road
Wilton, CT 06897
Phone: (203) 761-1113
✑ *www.runningtimes.com*

Marathon & Beyond—**"run longer, better, smarter"**

206 N. Randolph St., Suite 400
Champaign, IL 61820
Phone: (217) 359-9345
✑ *www.marathonandbeyond.com*

National Masters News

P.O. Box 1117
Orangevale, CA 95662
Phone: (916) 989-6667
✑ *www.nationalmastersnews.com*

Trail Runner—**"helps runners of all ages and abilities experience the outdoors and achieve a healthier lifestyle through off-road running"**

417 Main St., Unit N
Carbondale, CO 81623
Phone: (970) 704-1442
✐ *www.trailrunnermag.com*

UltraRunning—**"the voice of the ultrarunner"**

5825 W. Dry Creek Road
Healdsburg, CA 95448
Phone: (707) 431-9898
✐ *www.ultrarunning.com*

Track & Field News—**"the bible of the sport since 1948"**

2570 El Camino Real, Suite 606
Mountain View, CA 94040
Phone: (650) 948-8188
✐ *www.trackandfieldnews.com*

Books

If you enjoy reading about running, you're already got one of the best books out there—this one! But like all sports and hobbies, running has produced a deep and wide body of works. The running library includes books on training for particular events, health and injuries, the psychology of running, and the pure enjoyment of running. This list is not all-inclusive, but it includes classics by

Dr. George Sheehan, Bob Glover, Jeff Galloway, Amby Burfoot, and Joan Benoit Samuelson.

Two publishers that specialize in books on running and physical fitness are Rodale Press in Emmaus, Pennsylvania, and Human Kinetics Publications in Champaign, Illinois. Many of their titles are listed below. You can also research their selections online by going to *www.rodale.com* and *www.humankinetics.com*.

General Training and Inspiration

Battista, Garth, ed. *The Runner's Literary Companion: Great Stories and Poems About Running.* (Penguin USA, 1996)

Battista, Garth. *How Running Changed My Life: True Stories of the Power of Running.* (Breakaway Books, 2002)

Bingham, John. *No Need for Speed: A Beginner's Guide to the Joy of Running.* (Rodale, 2002)

Bloom, Marc. *Run With the Champions: Training Programs and Secrets of America's 50 Greatest Runners.* (Rodale, 2001)

Burfoot, Amby, ed. *Runner's World Complete Book of Running: Everything You Need to Know to Run for Fun, Fitness, and Competition.* (Rodale, 1997)

Burfoot, Amby. *The Principles of Running.* (Rodale, 1999)

Burfoot, Amby. *The Runner's Guide to the Meaning of Life: What 35 Years of Running Has Taught*

Me About Winning, Losing, Happiness, Humility, and the Human Heart. (Daybreak Books, 2000)

Burfoot, Amby. *Runner's World Complete Book of Beginning Running.* (Rodale, 2005)

Chase, Adam and Nancy Hobbs. *The Ultimate Guide to Trail Running.* (Lyons Press, 2001)

Couch, Jean. *The Runner's Yoga Book: A Balanced Approach to Fitness.* (Rodmell Press, 1990)

Craythorn, Dennis and Rich Hanna. *The Ultimate Runner's Journal: Your Daily Training Partner and Log.* (Marathon Publishing, 1998)

Daniels, Jack. *Daniels' Running Formula.* (Human Kinetics, 2004)

Ellis, Joe and Joe Henderson. *Running Injury-Free: How to Prevent, Treat, and Recover from Dozens of Painful Problems.* (Rodale, 1994)

Fishpool, Sean. *Beginner's Guide to Long-Distance Running.* (Barrons, 2005)

Galloway, Jeff. *Galloway's Book on Running.* (Shelter Publications, 1984)

Galloway, Jeff. *Jeff Galloway's Training Journal.* (Phidippides Publication, 1998)

Glover, Bob and Shelly-Lynn Florence Glover. *The Competitive Runner's Handbook: The Bestselling Guide to Running 5Ks Through Marathons.* (Penguin USA, 1999)

Glover, Bob. *The Runner's Handbook: The Best-Selling Classic Fitness Guide for Beginner and Intermediate Runners.* (Penguin USA, 1996)

Glover, Bob and Shelly-Lynn Florence Glover. *The Runner's Training Diary: For Fitness Runners and Competitive Racers.* (Penguin USA, 1997)

Henderson, Joe and Amby Burfoot. *Best Runs.* (Human Kinetics, 1998)

Henderson, Joe and Jeff Galloway. *Better Runs: 25 Years' Worth of Lessons for Running Faster and Farther.* (Human Kinetics, 1995)

Henderson, Joe and Hal Higdon. *Running 101.* (Human Kinetics, 2000)

Higdon, Hal. *Hal Higdon's How to Train: The Best Programs, Workouts, and Schedules for Runners of All Ages.* (Rodale, 1997)

Higdon, Hal. *Hal Higdon's Smart Running: Expert Advice on Training, Motivation, Injury Prevention, Nutrition, and Good Health for Runners of Any Age and Ability.* (Rodale, 1998)

Higdon, Hal. *Run Fast: How to Beat Your Best Time Every Time.* (Rodale, 2000)

Higdon, Hal. *Run Fast: How to Train for a 5-K or 10-K Race.* (Rodale, 1992)

Kowalchik, Claire. *The Complete Book of Running for Women.* (Pocket Books, 1999)

Lundgren, Chris. *Runner's World Guide to Running and Pregnancy.* (Rodale, 2003)

Lynch, Jerry and Warren A. Scott. *Running Within: A Guide to Mastering the Mind-Body-Spirit Connection for Ultimate Training and Racing.* (Human Kinetics, 1999)

MacNeil, Ian. *The Beginning Runner's Handbook: The Proven 13-Week Walk/Run Program.* (Greystone Publishing, 1999)

Martin, David E. and Peter N. Coe. *Better Training for Distance Runners.* (Human Kinetics, 1997)

McMillan, Greg and Juliana Risner. *Zap! You're a Runner.* (Road Runner Sports, 1999)

Nelson, Kevin. *The Runner's Book of Daily Inspiration: A Year of Motivation, Revelation, and Instruction.* (McGraw-Hill, 1999)

Noakes, Tim. *Lore of Running.* (Human Kinetics, 2002)

Noakes, Tim and Stephen Granger. *Running Injuries: How to Prevent and Overcome Them.* (Oxford University Press, 2003)

Poulin, Kirsten, Christina Flaxel, MD, and Stan Swartz. *Trail Running: From Novice to Master.* (Mountaineers Books, 2002)

Reese, Paul. *The Old Man and the Road: Reflections While Completing a Crossing of All 50 States on Foot at Age 80.* (Keokee Co. Publishing, 2000)

Runner's World Magazine. *Runner's World: Training Journal.* (Wiley, published annually)

Scott, Dagny. *Runner's World Complete Book of Women's Running: The Best Advice to Get Started, Stay Motivated, Lose Weight, Run Injury-Free, Be Safe, and Train for Any Distance.* (Rodale, 2000)

Sheehan, George. *Dr. George Sheehan on Getting Fit and Feeling Great: How to Feel Great 24 Hours a Day/Running and Being/This Running Life/ Three Volumes in One.* (Listen U.S.A. 1985)

Sheehan, George. *George Sheehan on Running to Win: How to Achieve the Physical, Mental & Spiritual Victories of Running.* (Rodale, 1994)

Sheehan, George. *Going the Distance: One Man's Journey to the End of His Life.* (Villard Books, 1996)

Sheehan, George. *Personal Best: The Foremost Philosopher of Fitness Shares Techniques and Tactics for Success and Self-Liberation.* (Rodale, 1992)

Sheehan, George. *Running and Being: The Total Experience.* (Second Wind II, 1998)

Svensson, Sharon L. *The Total Runner's Log: The Essential Training Tool for the Runner.* (Trimarket, 1998)

Weisenfeld, Murray and Barbara Burr. *The Runner's Repair Manual: A Complete Program for Diagnosing and Treating Your Foot, Leg and Back Problems.* (St. Martin's Press, 1981)

Will-Weber, Mark, ed. *The Quotable Runner: Great Moments of Wisdom, Inspiration, Wrongheartedness, and Humor.* (Breakaway Books, 1995)

Marathon Training

Bloch, Gordon Bakoulis. *How to Train for and Run Your Best Marathon.* (Fireside, 1993)

Galloway, Jeff. *Marathon!* (Phidippides Publications, 2000)

Griffin, Jane. *Nutrition for Marathon Running.* (Crowood Press, 2005)

Hanc, John and Grete Waitz. *The Essential Marathoner: A Concise Guide to the Race of Your Life.* (Lyons Press, 1996)

Henderson, Joe. *Marathon Training: The Proven 100-Day Program for Success.* (Human Kinetics, 1997)

Higdon, Hal. *Marathon: The Ultimate Training Guide.* (Rodale, 1999)

Nerurkar, Richard and Steve Cram. *Marathon Running: The Complete Training Guide.* (Lyons Press, 2001)

Pfitzinger, Pete and Scott Douglas. *Advanced Marathoning.* (Human Kinetics, 2001)

Whitsett, David A., Forrest A. Dolgener, and Tanjala Mabon Kole. *The Non-Runner's Marathon Trainer.* (McGraw-Hill, 1998)

Marathon History

Boeder, Robert B. *Beyond the Marathon: The Grand Slam of Trail Ultrarunning* (Old Mountain Press, 1996)

Connelly, Michael. *26 Miles to Boston: The Boston Marathon Experience from Hopkinton to Copley Square.* (The Lyons Press, 2003)

Derderian, Tom. *The Boston Marathon: A Century of Blood, Sweat, and Cheers.* (Triumph Books, 2003)

Derderian, Tom. *Boston Marathon: The First Century of the World's Premier Running Event.* (Human Kinetics, 1996)

Lonergan, Tom. *Heartbreak Hill: The Boston Marathon Thriller.* Fiction. (Writers Club Press, 2002)

Martin, David E. and Roger W. H. Gynn. *The Olympic Marathon.* (Human Kinetics, 2000)

Rubin, Ron. *Anything For A T-shirt: Fred Lebow And The New York City Marathon, The World's Greatest Footrace.* (Syracuse University Press, 2004)

Appendix C

Running Online

Since the first edition of this book was released back in 2002, the Web has exploded with new sites on running, from running barefoot to ultra-running. The sites included here are just a sampling of what's available online. If you search for something specific, like "running vacations," you're sure to tap into sites that seem custom-made for your interests.

A great place to begin your search is at *www .marathontraining.com*. Go to the site map, and then look under "Runner's Resources." There you will find a listing of useful sites that is continuously updated and added to. It includes general links, marathon training, online record-keeping, calendars, gear, and much more. The following annotated sites are some favorites as well.

General Sites

Cool Running—Race calendars, training tips, information on youth running; it's all here. *www.coolrunning.com*

Runners Web—A running and triathlon resource site. *www.runnersweb.com*

Road Runners Club of America—Over 700 clubs and 180,000 members throughout America. *www.rrca.org*

On the Run—Your online source for the long-distance running community. *www.ontherun. com*

Running Network—The most comprehensive source of information for grassroots runners online. *www.runningnetwork com*

Runner's World Magazine—It's not just a Web site for the magazine; it's a world of advice for runners. *www.runnersworld.com*

Running on the Web—A list of running-related sites. *http://sorrel.humboldt.edu/~rrw1/runweb .html*

Dr. Pribut's Sports Medicine Page—A site with lots of helpful sports medicine information. *www.drpribut.com*

Global Health and Fitness—Tells you everything you need to know to eat right, stay in shape, and feel great. *www.global-fitness.com*

Marathon Training Web Sites

State of the Art Marathon Training—Offers a wide range of running topics designed to meet the needs of the beginner to the advanced competitor. *www.marathontraining.com*

Hal Higdon On the Run—Provides advice from a foremost marathon competitor and trainer. *www.halhigdon.com*

Jeff Galloway's Marathon Training Program—Check out the official site from the guy who started a marathoning revolution. *www.jeffgalloway.com*

USA Fit—"Change your life" with helpful marathon tips. *www.usafit.com*

Association of International Marathons and Distance Races—Tap into the international running community here. *www.aims-association.org*

Ultra-Running

Ultra-Running Resource Site—Gives you information on every aspect of ultra-running. *www.ultrunr.com*

Official Web site of the Western States 100—A great site to look at to understand what's involved in an endurance run. *www.ws100.com*

American Ultra-Running Association—A resource for news and information on ultra-running in the United States. *www.americanultra.org*

Ultrarunning Online—Provides interesting articles and photos for ultra-runners. *www.ultrarunning.com*

Index

H

Half-marathon, training for, 155–56
Half-marathon training schedules, 156t
Hamstring stretches, 171, 172
Health benefits, 5
Health club, alternative to, 12
Heat-induced illnesses, 117–18
Heel
contact, 174
counter, 26
heights, 27
lift, 182, 194
notch, 26
slippage, 28
spurs, 187–88, 189
strike, 46
Heel-ball footstrike, 43, 46–47
High arch, 170
High-impact sports, 13, 105
Hill repeats, 136–37
Hip abductor strengthening, 196
Hot weather running, 115–19
HVGS (high voltage galvanic stimulation), 182, 194, 197
Hydrated, staying
marathon and, 233
options for, 33
pre-competition and, 72, 73
during run, 59
side effects of, 60
weather and, 115, 116
Hydrating/dehydrating fluids, 208–09
Hyer, Linda, 10
Hyponatremia, 73, 116, 208

I

Iliotibial band, 86
Iliotibial band (ITB) syndrome, 195–96
Indian Journal of Medical Research, 110
Indoors, running, 119–20
Injuries, avoiding, 21
Injuries, exercising the, 185
Injuries, foot/ankle
achilles tendonitis and, 180–82
ankle sprains and, 184–85
anterior ankle pain and, 185
athlete's foot and, 186–87
exercising an injury and, 185
guidelines for, 180
heel spurs and, 187–88, 189
neuroma pain and, 189–90
plantar fasciitis and, 187–89
ruptured achilles tendon and, 183–84
stretching and, 182
training modifications and, 182
Injuries, miscellaneous
compartment syndrome and, 192
iliotibial band (ITB) syndrome and, 195–96
medial shine splints and, 196–97
nonstress fracture and, 192
runner's knee and, 198–200
shin splints and, 192–94, 200
side stitches and, 200–201
soft tissue and, 192
stress fracture and, 192
Injuries, prevention of
achilles tendonitis, 168–69
arm movement and, 176
the basics of, 166–67
guide to shoes/foot problems and, 170
icing and, 167
medications and, 166
overstretching and, 172
plantar fasciitis and, 169
running shoes and, 167–70
stretching and, 170–72
treating inflammation and, 166–67
Injuries, risk of, 126–27
Interval workouts, 140–43

J

Joint flexibility, 8

THE EVERYTHING SERIES!

BUSINESS & PERSONAL FINANCE

Everything® Accounting Book
Everything® Budgeting Book, 2nd Ed.
Everything® Business Planning Book
Everything® Coaching and Mentoring Book, 2nd Ed.
Everything® Fundraising Book
Everything® Get Out of Debt Book
Everything® Grant Writing Book, 2nd Ed.
Everything® Guide to Buying Foreclosures
Everything® Guide to Fundraising, $15.95
Everything® Guide to Mortgages
Everything® Guide to Personal Finance for Single Mothers
Everything® Home-Based Business Book, 2nd Ed.
Everything® Homebuying Book, 3rd Ed., $15.95
Everything® Homeselling Book, 2nd Ed.
Everything® Human Resource Management Book
Everything® Improve Your Credit Book
Everything® Investing Book, 2nd Ed.
Everything® Landlording Book
Everything® Leadership Book, 2nd Ed.
Everything® Managing People Book, 2nd Ed.
Everything® Negotiating Book
Everything® Online Auctions Book
Everything® Online Business Book
Everything® Personal Finance Book
Everything® Personal Finance in Your 20s & 30s Book, 2nd Ed.
Everything® Personal Finance in Your 40s & 50s Book, $15.95
Everything® Project Management Book, 2nd Ed.
Everything® Real Estate Investing Book
Everything® Retirement Planning Book
Everything® Robert's Rules Book, $7.95
Everything® Selling Book
Everything® Start Your Own Business Book, 2nd Ed.
Everything® Wills & Estate Planning Book

COOKING

Everything® Barbecue Cookbook
Everything® Bartender's Book, 2nd Ed., $9.95
Everything® Calorie Counting Cookbook
Everything® Cheese Book
Everything® Chinese Cookbook
Everything® Classic Recipes Book
Everything® Cocktail Parties & Drinks Book
Everything® College Cookbook
Everything® Cooking for Baby and Toddler Book
Everything® Diabetes Cookbook
Everything® Easy Gourmet Cookbook
Everything® Fondue Cookbook
Everything® Food Allergy Cookbook, $15.95
Everything® Fondue Party Book
Everything® Gluten-Free Cookbook
Everything® Glycemic Index Cookbook
Everything® Grilling Cookbook
Everything® Healthy Cooking for Parties Book, $15.95
Everything® Holiday Cookbook
Everything® Indian Cookbook
Everything® Lactose-Free Cookbook
Everything® Low-Cholesterol Cookbook

Everything® Low-Fat High-Flavor Cookbook, 2nd Ed., $15.95
Everything® Low-Salt Cookbook
Everything® Meals for a Month Cookbook
Everything® Meals on a Budget Cookbook
Everything® Mediterranean Cookbook
Everything® Mexican Cookbook
Everything® No Trans Fat Cookbook
Everything® One-Pot Cookbook, 2nd Ed., $15.95
Everything® Organic Cooking for Baby & Toddler Book, $15.95
Everything® Pizza Cookbook
Everything® Quick Meals Cookbook, 2nd Ed., $15.95
Everything® Slow Cooker Cookbook
Everything® Slow Cooking for a Crowd Cookbook
Everything® Soup Cookbook
Everything® Stir-Fry Cookbook
Everything® Sugar-Free Cookbook
Everything® Tapas and Small Plates Cookbook
Everything® Tex-Mex Cookbook
Everything® Thai Cookbook
Everything® Vegetarian Cookbook
Everything® Whole-Grain, High-Fiber Cookbook
Everything® Wild Game Cookbook
Everything® Wine Book, 2nd Ed.

GAMES

Everything® 15-Minute Sudoku Book, $9.95
Everything® 30-Minute Sudoku Book, $9.95
Everything® Bible Crosswords Book, $9.95
Everything® Blackjack Strategy Book
Everything® Brain Strain Book, $9.95
Everything® Bridge Book
Everything® Card Games Book
Everything® Card Tricks Book, $9.95
Everything® Casino Gambling Book, 2nd Ed.
Everything® Chess Basics Book
Everything® Christmas Crosswords Book, $9.95
Everything® Craps Strategy Book
Everything® Crossword and Puzzle Book
Everything® Crosswords and Puzzles for Quote Lovers Book, $9.95
Everything® Crossword Challenge Book
Everything® Crosswords for the Beach Book, $9.95
Everything® Cryptic Crosswords Book, $9.95
Everything® Cryptograms Book, $9.95
Everything® Easy Crosswords Book
Everything® Easy Kakuro Book, $9.95
Everything® Easy Large-Print Crosswords Book
Everything® Games Book, 2nd Ed.
Everything® Giant Book of Crosswords
Everything® Giant Sudoku Book, $9.95
Everything® Giant Word Search Book
Everything® Kakuro Challenge Book, $9.95
Everything® Large-Print Crossword Challenge Book
Everything® Large-Print Crosswords Book
Everything® Large-Print Travel Crosswords Book
Everything® Lateral Thinking Puzzles Book, $9.95
Everything® Literary Crosswords Book, $9.95
Everything® Mazes Book
Everything® Memory Booster Puzzles Book, $9.95

Everything® Movie Crosswords Book, $9.95
Everything® Music Crosswords Book, $9.95
Everything® Online Poker Book
Everything® Pencil Puzzles Book, $9.95
Everything® Poker Strategy Book
Everything® Pool & Billiards Book
Everything® Puzzles for Commuters Book, $9.95
Everything® Puzzles for Dog Lovers Book, $9.95
Everything® Sports Crosswords Book, $9.95
Everything® Test Your IQ Book, $9.95
Everything® Texas Hold 'Em Book, $9.95
Everything® Travel Crosswords Book, $9.95
Everything® Travel Mazes Book, $9.95
Everything® Travel Word Search Book, $9.95
Everything® TV Crosswords Book, $9.95
Everything® Word Games Challenge Book
Everything® Word Scramble Book
Everything® Word Search Book

HEALTH

Everything® Alzheimer's Book
Everything® Diabetes Book
Everything® First Aid Book, $9.95
Everything® Green Living Book
Everything® Health Guide to Addiction and Recovery
Everything® Health Guide to Adult Bipolar Disorder
Everything® Health Guide to Arthritis
Everything® Health Guide to Controlling Anxiety
Everything® Health Guide to Depression
Everything® Health Guide to Diabetes, 2nd Ed.
Everything® Health Guide to Fibromyalgia
Everything® Health Guide to Menopause, 2nd Ed.
Everything® Health Guide to Migraines
Everything® Health Guide to Multiple Sclerosis
Everything® Health Guide to OCD
Everything® Health Guide to PMS
Everything® Health Guide to Postpartum Care
Everything® Health Guide to Thyroid Disease
Everything® Hypnosis Book
Everything® Low Cholesterol Book
Everything® Menopause Book
Everything® Nutrition Book
Everything® Reflexology Book
Everything® Stress Management Book
Everything® Superfoods Book, $15.95

HISTORY

Everything® American Government Book
Everything® American History Book, 2nd Ed.
Everything® American Revolution Book, $15.95
Everything® Civil War Book
Everything® Freemasons Book
Everything® Irish History & Heritage Book
Everything® World War II Book, 2nd Ed.

HOBBIES

Everything® Candlemaking Book
Everything® Cartooning Book
Everything® Coin Collecting Book
Everything® Digital Photography Book, 2nd Ed.

Everything® Drawing Book
Everything® Family Tree Book, 2nd Ed.
Everything® Guide to Online Genealogy, $15.95
Everything® Knitting Book
Everything® Knots Book
Everything® Photography Book
Everything® Quilting Book
Everything® Sewing Book
Everything® Soapmaking Book, 2nd Ed.
Everything® Woodworking Book

HOME IMPROVEMENT

Everything® Feng Shui Book
Everything® Feng Shui Decluttering Book, $9.95
Everything® Fix-It Book
Everything® Green Living Book
Everything® Home Decorating Book
Everything® Home Storage Solutions Book
Everything® Homebuilding Book
Everything® Organize Your Home Book, 2nd Ed.

KIDS' BOOKS

All titles are $7.95
Everything® Fairy Tales Book, $14.95
Everything® Kids' Animal Puzzle & Activity Book
Everything® Kids' Astronomy Book
Everything® Kids' Baseball Book, 5th Ed.
Everything® Kids' Bible Trivia Book
Everything® Kids' Bugs Book
Everything® Kids' Cars and Trucks Puzzle and Activity Book
Everything® Kids' Christmas Puzzle & Activity Book
Everything® Kids' Connect the Dots
Puzzle and Activity Book
Everything® Kids' Cookbook, 2nd Ed.
Everything® Kids' Crazy Puzzles Book
Everything® Kids' Dinosaurs Book
Everything® Kids' Dragons Puzzle and Activity Book
Everything® Kids' Environment Book $7.95
Everything® Kids' Fairies Puzzle and Activity Book
Everything® Kids' First Spanish Puzzle and Activity Book
Everything® Kids' Football Book
Everything® Kids' Geography Book
Everything® Kids' Gross Cookbook
Everything® Kids' Gross Hidden Pictures Book
Everything® Kids' Gross Jokes Book
Everything® Kids' Gross Mazes Book
Everything® Kids' Gross Puzzle & Activity Book
Everything® Kids' Halloween Puzzle & Activity Book
Everything® Kids' Hanukkah Puzzle and Activity Book
Everything® Kids' Hidden Pictures Book
Everything® Kids' Horses Book
Everything® Kids' Joke Book
Everything® Kids' Knock Knock Book
Everything® Kids' Learning French Book
Everything® Kids' Learning Spanish Book
Everything® Kids' Magical Science Experiments Book
Everything® Kids' Math Puzzles Book
Everything® Kids' Mazes Book
Everything® Kids' Money Book, 2nd Ed.
Everything® Kids' Mummies, Pharaoh's, and Pyramids Puzzle and Activity Book
Everything® Kids' Nature Book
Everything® Kids' Pirates Puzzle and Activity Book
Everything® Kids' Presidents Book
Everything® Kids' Princess Puzzle and Activity Book
Everything® Kids' Puzzle Book

Everything® Kids' Racecars Puzzle and Activity Book
Everything® Kids' Riddles & Brain Teasers Book
Everything® Kids' Science Experiments Book
Everything® Kids' Sharks Book
Everything® Kids' Soccer Book
Everything® Kids' Spelling Book
Everything® Kids' Spies Puzzle and Activity Book
Everything® Kids' States Book
Everything® Kids' Travel Activity Book
Everything® Kids' Word Search Puzzle and Activity Book

LANGUAGE

Everything® Conversational Japanese Book with CD, $19.95
Everything® French Grammar Book
Everything® French Phrase Book, $9.95
Everything® French Verb Book, $9.95
Everything® German Phrase Book, $9.95
Everything® German Practice Book with CD, $19.95
Everything® Inglés Book
Everything® Intermediate Spanish Book with CD, $19.95
Everything® Italian Phrase Book, $9.95
Everything® Italian Practice Book with CD, $19.95
Everything® Learning Brazilian Portuguese Book with CD, $19.95
Everything® Learning French Book with CD, 2nd Ed., $19.95
Everything® Learning German Book
Everything® Learning Italian Book
Everything® Learning Latin Book
Everything® Learning Russian Book with CD, $19.95
Everything® Learning Spanish Book
Everything® Learning Spanish Book with CD, 2nd Ed., $19.95
Everything® Russian Practice Book with CD, $19.95
Everything® Sign Language Book, $15.95
Everything® Spanish Grammar Book
Everything® Spanish Phrase Book, $9.95
Everything® Spanish Practice Book with CD, $19.95
Everything® Spanish Verb Book, $9.95
Everything® Speaking Mandarin Chinese Book with CD, $19.95

MUSIC

Everything® Bass Guitar Book with CD, $19.95
Everything® Drums Book with CD, $19.95
Everything® Guitar Book with CD, 2nd Ed., $19.95
Everything® Guitar Chords Book with CD, $19.95
Everything® Guitar Scales Book with CD, $19.95
Everything® Harmonica Book with CD, $15.95
Everything® Home Recording Book
Everything® Music Theory Book with CD, $19.95
Everything® Reading Music Book with CD, $19.95
Everything® Rock & Blues Guitar Book with CD, $19.95
Everything® Rock & Blues Piano Book with CD, $19.95
Everything® Rock Drums Book with CD, $19.95
Everything® Singing Book with CD, $19.95
Everything® Songwriting Book

NEW AGE

Everything® Astrology Book, 2nd Ed.
Everything® Birthday Personology Book
Everything® Celtic Wisdom Book, $15.95
Everything® Dreams Book, 2nd Ed.
Everything® Law of Attraction Book, $15.95
Everything® Love Signs Book, $9.95
Everything® Love Spells Book, $9.95
Everything® Palmistry Book
Everything® Psychic Book
Everything® Reiki Book

Everything® Sex Signs Book, $9.95
Everything® Spells & Charms Book, 2nd Ed.
Everything® Tarot Book, 2nd Ed.
Everything® Toltec Wisdom Book
Everything® Wicca & Witchcraft Book, 2nd Ed.

PARENTING

Everything® Baby Names Book, 2nd Ed.
Everything® Baby Shower Book, 2nd Ed.
Everything® Baby Sign Language Book with DVD
Everything® Baby's First Year Book
Everything® Birthing Book
Everything® Breastfeeding Book
Everything® Father-to-Be Book
Everything® Father's First Year Book
Everything® Get Ready for Baby Book, 2nd Ed.
Everything® Get Your Baby to Sleep Book, $9.95
Everything® Getting Pregnant Book
Everything® Guide to Pregnancy Over 35
Everything® Guide to Raising a One-Year-Old
Everything® Guide to Raising a Two-Year-Old
Everything® Guide to Raising Adolescent Boys
Everything® Guide to Raising Adolescent Girls
Everything® Mother's First Year Book
Everything® Parent's Guide to Childhood Illnesses
Everything® Parent's Guide to Children and Divorce
Everything® Parent's Guide to Children with ADD/ADHD
Everything® Parent's Guide to Children with Asperger's Syndrome
Everything® Parent's Guide to Children with Anxiety
Everything® Parent's Guide to Children with Asthma
Everything® Parent's Guide to Children with Autism
Everything® Parent's Guide to Children with Bipolar Disorder
Everything® Parent's Guide to Children with Depression
Everything® Parent's Guide to Children with Dyslexia
Everything® Parent's Guide to Children with Juvenile Diabetes
Everything® Parent's Guide to Children with OCD
Everything® Parent's Guide to Positive Discipline
Everything® Parent's Guide to Raising Boys
Everything® Parent's Guide to Raising Girls
Everything® Parent's Guide to Raising Siblings
Everything® Parent's Guide to Raising Your Adopted Child
Everything® Parent's Guide to Sensory Integration Disorder
Everything® Parent's Guide to Tantrums
Everything® Parent's Guide to the Strong-Willed Child
Everything® Parenting a Teenager Book
Everything® Potty Training Book, $9.95
Everything® Pregnancy Book, 3rd Ed.
Everything® Pregnancy Fitness Book
Everything® Pregnancy Nutrition Book
Everything® Pregnancy Organizer, 2nd Ed., $16.95
Everything® Toddler Activities Book
Everything® Toddler Book
Everything® Tween Book
Everything® Twins, Triplets, and More Book

PETS

Everything® Aquarium Book
Everything® Boxer Book
Everything® Cat Book, 2nd Ed.
Everything® Chihuahua Book
Everything® Cooking for Dogs Book
Everything® Dachshund Book
Everything® Dog Book, 2nd Ed.
Everything® Dog Grooming Book

Everything® Dog Obedience Book
Everything® Dog Owner's Organizer, $16.95
Everything® Dog Training and Tricks Book
Everything® German Shepherd Book
Everything® Golden Retriever Book
Everything® Horse Book, 2nd Ed., $15.95
Everything® Horse Care Book
Everything® Horseback Riding Book
Everything® Labrador Retriever Book
Everything® Poodle Book
Everything® Pug Book
Everything® Puppy Book
Everything® Small Dogs Book
Everything® Tropical Fish Book
Everything® Yorkshire Terrier Book

REFERENCE

Everything® American Presidents Book
Everything® Blogging Book
Everything® Build Your Vocabulary Book, $9.95
Everything® Car Care Book
Everything® Classical Mythology Book
Everything® Da Vinci Book
Everything® Einstein Book
Everything® Enneagram Book
Everything® Etiquette Book, 2nd Ed.
Everything® Family Christmas Book, $15.95
Everything® Guide to Divorce, 2nd Ed., $15.95
Everything® Guide to C. S. Lewis & Narnia
Everything® Guide to Edgar Allan Poe
Everything® Guide to Understanding Philosophy
Everything® Inventions and Patents Book
Everything® Jacqueline Kennedy Onassis Book
Everything® John F. Kennedy Book
Everything® Mafia Book
Everything® Martin Luther King Jr. Book
Everything® Pirates Book
Everything® Private Investigation Book
Everything® Psychology Book
Everything® Public Speaking Book, $9.95
Everything® Shakespeare Book, 2nd Ed.

RELIGION

Everything® Angels Book
Everything® Bible Book
Everything® Bible Study Book with CD, $19.95
Everything® Buddhism Book
Everything® Catholicism Book
Everything® Christianity Book
Everything® Gnostic Gospels Book
Everything® Hinduism Book, $15.95
Everything® History of the Bible Book
Everything® Jesus Book
Everything® Jewish History & Heritage Book
Everything® Judaism Book
Everything® Kabbalah Book
Everything® Koran Book
Everything® Mary Book
Everything® Mary Magdalene Book
Everything® Prayer Book

Everything® Saints Book, 2nd Ed.
Everything® Torah Book
Everything® Understanding Islam Book
Everything® Women of the Bible Book
Everything® World's Religions Book

SCHOOL & CAREERS

Everything® Career Tests Book
Everything® College Major Test Book
Everything® College Survival Book, 2nd Ed.
Everything® Cover Letter Book, 2nd Ed.
Everything® Filmmaking Book
Everything® Get-a-Job Book, 2nd Ed.
Everything® Guide to Being a Paralegal
Everything® Guide to Being a Personal Trainer
Everything® Guide to Being a Real Estate Agent
Everything® Guide to Being a Sales Rep
Everything® Guide to Being an Event Planner
Everything® Guide to Careers in Health Care
Everything® Guide to Careers in Law Enforcement
Everything® Guide to Government Jobs
Everything® Guide to Starting and Running a Catering Business
Everything® Guide to Starting and Running a Restaurant
Everything® Guide to Starting and Running a Retail Store
Everything® Job Interview Book, 2nd Ed.
Everything® New Nurse Book
Everything® New Teacher Book
Everything® Paying for College Book
Everything® Practice Interview Book
Everything® Resume Book, 3rd Ed.
Everything® Study Book

SELF-HELP

Everything® Body Language Book
Everything® Dating Book, 2nd Ed.
Everything® Great Sex Book
Everything® Guide to Caring for Aging Parents, $15.95
Everything® Self-Esteem Book
Everything® Self-Hypnosis Book, $9.95
Everything® Tantric Sex Book

SPORTS & FITNESS

Everything® Easy Fitness Book
Everything® Fishing Book
Everything® Guide to Weight Training, $15.95
Everything® Krav Maga for Fitness Book
Everything® Running Book, 2nd Ed.
Everything® Triathlon Training Book, $15.95

TRAVEL

Everything® Family Guide to Coastal Florida
Everything® Family Guide to Cruise Vacations
Everything® Family Guide to Hawaii
Everything® Family Guide to Las Vegas, 2nd Ed.
Everything® Family Guide to Mexico
Everything® Family Guide to New England, 2nd Ed.

Everything® Family Guide to New York City, 3rd Ed.
Everything® Family Guide to Northern California and Lake Tahoe
Everything® Family Guide to RV Travel & Campgrounds
Everything® Family Guide to the Caribbean
Everything® Family Guide to the Disneyland® Resort, California Adventure®, Universal Studios®, and the Anaheim Area, 2nd Ed.
Everything® Family Guide to the Walt Disney World Resort®, Universal Studios®, and Greater Orlando, 5th Ed.
Everything® Family Guide to Timeshares
Everything® Family Guide to Washington D.C., 2nd Ed.

WEDDINGS

Everything® Bachelorette Party Book, $9.95
Everything® Bridesmaid Book, $9.95
Everything® Destination Wedding Book
Everything® Father of the Bride Book, $9.95
Everything® Green Wedding Book, $15.95
Everything® Groom Book, $9.95
Everything® Jewish Wedding Book, 2nd Ed., $15.95
Everything® Mother of the Bride Book, $9.95
Everything® Outdoor Wedding Book
Everything® Wedding Book, 3rd Ed.
Everything® Wedding Checklist, $9.95
Everything® Wedding Etiquette Book, $9.95
Everything® Wedding Organizer, 2nd Ed., $16.95
Everything® Wedding Shower Book, $9.95
Everything® Wedding Vows Book, 3rd Ed., $9.95
Everything® Wedding Workout Book
Everything® Weddings on a Budget Book, 2nd Ed., $9.95

WRITING

Everything® Creative Writing Book
Everything® Get Published Book, 2nd Ed.
Everything® Grammar and Style Book, 2nd Ed.
Everything® Guide to Magazine Writing
Everything® Guide to Writing a Book Proposal
Everything® Guide to Writing a Novel
Everything® Guide to Writing Children's Books
Everything® Guide to Writing Copy
Everything® Guide to Writing Graphic Novels
Everything® Guide to Writing Research Papers
Everything® Guide to Writing a Romance Novel, $15.95
Everything® Improve Your Writing Book, 2nd Ed.
Everything® Writing Poetry Book